Eat Well for a Healthy Menopause

Eat Well for a Healthy Menopause

The Low-Fat, High-Nutrition Guide

Elaine Moquette-Magee, M.P.H., R.D.

John Wiley & Sons, Inc.

New York • Chichester • Brisbane • Toronto • Singapore

Copyright © 1996 by Elaine Moquette-Magee
Published by John Wiley & Sons, Inc.

Composition, editorial services, and production management provided by Professional Book Center, Denver, Colorado.

The information contained in this book is not intended to serve as a replacement for the advice of a physician. Any use of the information set forth in this book is at the reader's discretion. The author and publisher specifically disclaim any and all liability arising directly or indirectly from the use or application of any information contained in this book.

Library of Congress Cataloging-in-Publication Data
Moquette-Magee, Elaine.
    Eat well for a healthy menopause : the low-fat, high-nutrition
  guide / Elaine Moquette-Magee.
      p. cm.
    Includes bibliographical references and index.
    ISBN 0-471-12250-5 (pbk. : alk.paper)
    ISBN 0-471-19360-7 (mass market)
    1. Middle aged women---Nutrition. 2. Middle aged women---Health and
  hygiene. 3. Menopause---Nutritional aspects. I. Title.
  RA778.M756 1996
  618.2'082---dc20   95-41711

Printed in the United States of America

10 9 8 7 6 5 4 3 2 1

*To Nesly Moquette, the best mother
(and grandma) I could ever hope for.
Mom—this one's for you!*

ACKNOWLEDGMENTS

I first need to thank Sue Gillespie, my nurse practitioner friend who urged me to write a book about diet and menopause. I can honestly say if not for her, the thought would never have crossed my mind (at the time she first mentioned it to me, I was pregnant with my second daughter, and pretty much the last thing on my mind was menopause).

I also need to thank my tried and true agent, Laurie Harper, whose belief in me and this book got me through the tough times (and there were a few). I would also like to thank my editor, Judith McCarthy, for her brilliant work on the book.

Lastly, I would especially like to thank all the researchers who kindly took time out of their very busy schedules to answer questions or review various chapters of the book. Your comments and support were invaluable:

Jim Anderson, M.D., Professor of Medicine and Clinical Nutrition, VA Medical Center, Lexington, Kentucky

John Anderson, Ph.D., Professor of Nutrition, School of Public Health, University of North Carolina, Chapel Hill

Sue Cummings, M.S., R.D., Massachusetts General Hospital

Dr. James Duke and Dr. Stephen Beckstrom-Sternberg of the USDA Agricultural Research Service

Suzanne Murphy, Ph.D., R.D., Department of Nutritional Sciences, University of California, Berkeley

Dr. Simin Meydani, Human Nutrition Research Center on Aging, Tufts University, Massachusetts

Mindy Kurzer, Ph.D., University of Minnesota

And two prominent researchers who supported the chapters they reviewed but because of their positions in government and a university preferred to remain anonymous.

CONTENTS

INTRODUCTION

If you are reading this book, you probably have entered, or are about to enter, menopause. In times past, many women thought it was safe to eat anything they wanted at this time of life. They thought that when they turned 50, they could pass "GO," collect $200, and abandon any previous nutritional/dietary precautions. After all, the womb is retired and the need for iron decreases as soon as your period terminates, right? Wrong. For what we now know is that when you hit menopause, you are entering one of the most nutritionally challenging times of your life.

During menopause, a woman's need for certain nutrients increases. At the same time, she requires fewer total calories. That's the challenge: to eat smarter to maintain and even improve your health during a physically and emotionally turbulent time in your life. Fortunately, the science of nutrition is up to this challenge. In fact, the right diet can help:

- Relieve common menopausal discomforts.
- Keep off excess body fat.
- Maximize your body's absorption of vital nutrients.
- Maintain bowel regularity and comfort.
- Preserve as much of your bone mass as possible.
- Postpone or lessen the natural effects of aging.

The new information we have on good nutrition during menopause can make all your years after 50 more enjoyable—and you may live longer to boot. A healthy diet can improve both the quality and the quantity of your life at any age. Think about it. Today many 50-year-old women have a good 30 to 40 years left to live and *enjoy*. Living into your eighties can mean celebrating 20 wonderful years after retirement, watching your grandchildren grow up, and even seeing them graduate from college.

Our society refers to menopause as the "change of life." During this change, most women will be offered assorted prescriptions from everything medical science has to offer, to help us feel as comfortable as possible. But can diet prepare our bodies for this impending battle of the hormones? Can it help us while we're actively engaged in the battle? Can it help minimize wounds or scars? Yes, yes, and yes. It even makes good sense to start eating for a healthy menopause *before* you begin experiencing symptoms. This will give your body a head start and assure you peak nutrient stores and a lean physique when the change finally hits.

1

Eating during and after menopause is reminiscent of "eating for two" during pregnancy because, during this phase of our lives, the *nutrient density* of your diet becomes crucial. Around menopause and beyond, your daily requirements of certain vitamins and minerals *increase* due to a decrease in the absorption of vitamins and minerals in the intestinal tract. Also, major organs may become less efficient than they once were. At the same time, your caloric needs gradually *decrease* due to a lower metabolic rate and a lifestyle that tends to be less active. So you have to get *more* of many nutrients with *fewer* calories.

Some of the trials of menopause and beyond result from the natural process of aging. Most women begin to notice the effects of aging at about 30, but the process really kicks into high gear after menopause. In essence, our female hormones no longer help protect us from the human inevitability of aging. But just as harmful dietary and other lifestyle habits—such as smoking, overeating, excessive alcohol consumption, too much exposure to the sun, and so on—can *increase* the impact of age on our body, we can also adopt good habits to *slow* the aging process and *lessen* its effects.

I've encapsuled all the healthy nutritional practices you'll need into ten simple guidelines. To emphasize their importance, I've named them "the 10 Diet Commandments for a healthy menopause."

1. Eat at least one phytoestrogen-rich food every day.
2. Eat at least one boron-rich food every day.
3. Limit your intake of caffeine, soft drinks, and alcohol—and drink plenty of water.
4. Eat about 150 percent of the RDA for the vitamins and minerals you need more of as you age.
5. Eat many small meals throughout the day, and eat light at night.
6. Eat at least two calcium-rich foods every day, preferably ones also high in vitamin D.
7. Eat several antioxidant-rich foods every day.
8. Eat no more than 20 to 25 percent of your calories from fat.
9. Eat 20 to 30 grams of fiber every day, from a variety of different foods.
10. Limit your intake of sodium and sugar.

How do these 10 Diet Commandments help? Following these rules can make your menopause and later life healthier and more enjoyable by helping to:

• Alleviate the discomforts and common symptoms of menopause, whether they're followed in addition to or instead of hormone replacement therapy.

- Minimize the risks associated with hormone replacement therapy.
- Lessen or delay the discomforts and symptoms of the natural aging process.

WHY IS THIS BOOK NECESSARY?

You are probably aware of the multitude of books available today on menopause. But, shockingly, only a few of these discuss the effects of *diet* on menopause—and the few that do only skim the surface. Unfortunately, many of these books have been written by medical doctors who generally do not have training or practical experience in diet and nutrition. Also, it is only recent research that has provided significant evidence that diet can influence our hormonal balance and the resultant discomforts. This revolutionary idea means that diet can not only make you healthier, it may also be able to help make you more comfortable during menopause.

In order to help you actually use this new information, I'll not only explain *why* the nutritional guidelines set forth in the 10 Diet Commandments are necessary, but also show you *how* to meet them in your daily life. I'll also help you figure out how your current diet compares to the ideal diet, which follows the 10 Diet Commandments. For example, I don't find it effective simply to tell you to "eat more fiber." You need to know that you should eat 20 to 30 grams or more of fiber a day; what the highest-fiber foods are and exactly how much fiber they contain; and how to get the most fiber with the least amount of fat, calories, and inconvenience.

Moreover, the problem with general dietary guidelines is that we read them independent of each other. So when we try to combine them, making decisions about food can get complicated, to say the least. Do you choose more calcium over fewer calories? Do you worry more about fat or fiber? Do you become vehement about certain vitamins?

Eat Well for a Healthy Menopause pulls together all the most up-to-date information on all the critical health and dietary topics, and condenses everything into the 10 Diet Commandments. It provides practical tips, easy food tables, and quick, delicious recipes to get you started on heeding the 10 Diet Commandments, so you can begin to feel better than ever!

BACK TO BASICS: VARIETY AND BALANCE

Throughout this book, you'll notice that I continuously emphasize two basic nutrition concepts: variety and balance. These old-fashioned ideas are central to any healthy diet.

Too many of us—health professionals and consumers alike—have tried to find easy answers to the challenge of healthy eating by isolating different components of our diet: calcium's effect on osteoporosis, sodium's effect on hypertension, or saturated fat's effect on heart disease. Perhaps we who are health professionals and researchers have made the mistake of trying to answer questions about one disease with a one-nutrient answer. The truth is, the more we know about the causes and prevention of chronic diseases, the more apparent it becomes that there are *many* dietary factors that play a role in good health. That understanding leads us to a more balanced, complete view of health and disease—which brings us back to using food rather than pills to get our essential nutrients in nature-made combinations.

For example, eating fruits and vegetables has long been associated with a lower risk for almost every chronic disease, especially cancer. So researchers have been trying to isolate and test the effects of the various helpful components in fruits and vegetables, such as beta-carotene, vitamin C, and a handful of nutrients called phytochemicals. But when all is said and done, there are bound to be many other helpful components that we still don't understand. Further, their protective action is likely to result, not so much from the individual effects of each component, but from the way they work together.

This is why my 10 Diet Commandments emphasize *food habits* when possible rather than *nutrient levels*. In my estimation, all the new information becoming available about such food components as boron, antioxidants, lignans, phytochemicals, chemopreventive agents, fiber, and others leads us to the importance of balance: a diet that avoids excesses in fat and empty calories like sugar, but is richer in fruits, vegetables, and grains.

HEALTH AND ENJOYMENT: THE QUEST TO LOWER FAT

I've written a few books promoting the health merits and practicality of—as well as the potential enjoyment to be gained from—a low-fat diet. Not a very, very low-fat diet, but a fairly low-fat diet. Because while I believe in maximizing health, I also believe in enjoying life, which includes enjoying food. I find it much easier—and therefore more realistic—to lighten up traditional and favorite recipes toward the goal of consuming only 20 to 30 percent of your calories from fat, compared to the more extreme goal of consuming only 10 percent of your calories from fat that some health professionals advocate. And I can't forget something I once read that made a lot of sense: Deprivation feeds obsession. Therefore, I can't recommend a diet that would make you feel deprived and unsatisfied.

A moderately low-fat diet, however, is a cornerstone to healthful eating. Lowering the fat in your diet can actually improve your nutrient density. For example, when you switch from whole to nonfat or 1% low-fat milk, the amount of calcium and magnesium you get increases. And when you choose leaner cuts of red meat and pork, you get more protein and vitamin B-12 per ounce, not less.

WHERE DO WE GO FROM HERE?

If I sound a little wishy-washy at times in the chapters to come, softening statements with disclaimers like "may be protective," "possibly contributes," "preliminary evidence suggests," and "some experts believe," it's because research on nutrition's effects on menopause, aging, and disease prevention is still relatively new. As a result, we don't always have definitive data on which to base absolute opinions. However, all the nutritional advice given in this book is *natural.* That is, my recommendations are grounded in established dietary truths concerning the value of food. You certainly can't go wrong following the advice given here. While there are still some unanswered questions about dietary estrogen, the potential risks of hormone replacement therapy, and the effects of antioxidants on disease, many leading researchers agree that there is enough information to make some common-sense suggestions that will start helping women like you *now.* And that's what this book is all about.

HOW TO USE THIS BOOK

This book is filled to the brim with information that will help you achieve a higher level of health during menopause and beyond. Many of the chapters deal with subject matter that could easily comprise an entire book. So if you feel overwhelmed at times, you're not alone. I was immersed in the issues and research for an entire year. But what kept me sane and focused through the conception and delivery of this book was the organizing structure of the 10 Diet Commandments. So just remember that all the information contained herein will always lead you back to that structural framework.

Part One provides a perspective on the physiological changes a woman undergoes as she matures. Chapter 1 tells you (briefly) what you need to know about the medical aspects of menopause, while chapter 2 examines whether or not you should take hormones during and/or after menopause.

Part Two explains how diet can make you feel better during menopause and beyond. Chapter 3 describes how what and when you eat can alleviate some of the discomforts of menopause. Chapters 4, 5, and 6 introduce the first five Diet Commandments, with suggestions for acquiring estrogen from natural sources and for maintaining your youth and having more energy by taking in the right nutrients.

Disease prevention through proper diet is the topic of Part Three, which introduces the second five Diet Commandments. Chapter 7 investigates calcium and osteoporosis while chapter 8 explores the twin concerns of cancer and heart disease.

Part Four details how to follow the 10 Diet Commandments. Chapter 9 offers tips and advice on making each Diet Commandment part of your daily routine. And chapter 10 presents exercises designed to help you evaluate your current diet against each of the 10 Diet Commandments.

Finally, appendix A provides additional detailed information (in tabular format) on food sources of various nutrients, and appendix B offers a number of very tasty and healthy recipes.

If you find yourself feeling overloaded at any point while reading this book, *stop*. Reread the 10 Diet Commandments. Find calm and resolve in these ten simple steps to feeling better and staying healthier. The book will be there waiting for you when you're ready to dive in again. Best of health to you during menopause and beyond!

PART ONE

HOW MENOPAUSE AFFECTS YOUR BODY

1

MENOPAUSE, MEDICALLY SPEAKING

by Sue Gillespie, R.N.M.S., N.P., and Carol Wysham, M.D.

Menopause is one of the *transitional* phases of life through which all women pass. It can, however, mean different things to different women, in both physical and emotional terms. Each woman's journey is unique. For some women, menopause is only a flutter in their biological and emotional rhythms; for others, the change may be incredibly pronounced, an all-consuming passage causing tremendous upheaval in their lives.

The most difficult time for most women seems to be the period right before menopause. However, this period, called **perimenopause,** can also be a time of empowerment for many women, a time in which they recognize the possibilities for self-determination and self-responsibility, a time when they begin to realize that they do have some control and power over their own life—as part of and apart from the many roles they have heretofore been living.

A century ago, an American woman's life span was approximately 49 years, which meant that few women lived long beyond their childbearing years. In contrast, today the average American woman lives well into her eighth decade. In fact, more women will experience menopause today than at any other point in history.

Unfortunately, though, this common life experience for over half the world's population is not as well understood as it might—and should—be. So before you read about how to eat right during menopause, we'll first provide a brief overview of just what menopause really is.

LET'S GET PHYSICAL

Menopause refers to the end of all menstrual bleeding. Another term you may hear is the **climacteric,** which refers to the total transition period of declining fertility. The climacteric may take 15 to 20 years and is usually experienced from age 35 to age 55. These two terms are sometimes mistakenly used synonymously.

Some women experience menopause slowly, with gradually increasing signs of estrogen withdrawal. Others experience an abrupt stoppage in their menstrual cycling, with either no symptoms or with significant symptoms. If you have had a hysterectomy that included the removal of your ovaries, you have already experienced an abrupt stoppage in your cycle as well as an abrupt withdrawal from your own natural estrogen. This is called **surgical menopause.** Without some type of estrogen replacement, a woman experiencing surgical menopause is usually very uncomfortable, with symptoms (described later in this chapter) that can be severe.

Most women stop menstruating between the ages of 48 and 52, although there are those who will stop during their late thirties or early forties. At the other end of the spectrum (and much to their dismay), some women will continue with some natural monthly cycling (as opposed to cycling brought on by hormone replacement therapy) into their mid- to late fifties. And in case you were wondering, there is no correlation between the onset of **menarche** (when we start our periods) and the onset of menopause. Just because you started menstruating early (or late) doesn't mean you'll stop early (or late).

Although a women's endocrine system and the hormonal regulation of her monthly cycle seems quite complicated, a basic understanding of these natural processes will help in understanding what occurs when the monthly cycle begins to change.

HORMONES AND NEUROTRANSMITTERS

The **hypothalamus** is the brain-nerve link to hormone production. It puts out releasing hormones, takes in messages from our senses, and helps control many bodily functions, including control of the menstrual cycle. The **pituitary gland** lies directly beneath the hypothalamus (adjacent to the brain), and secretes hormones that stimulate and regulate other glands and organs. Both the hypothalamus and pituitary gland are considered master glands. The **thyroid gland,** the **adrenal glands,** the **pancreas,** and the **female reproductive system** (including the **uterus** and the **ovaries**) also play a primary part in the regulation of many of our body's functions.

Working in tandem with the organs and glands of the endocrine system are **hormones** and **neurotransmitters.** Hormones are chemical substances produced in one part of the body and carried by the blood to another part in order to fulfill a specific purpose or control a body process. Our body is like a puzzle with a zillion pieces. Amazingly enough, as the hormone "puzzle piece" travels around the body in our bloodstream, it is ultimately recognized by a receptor on one of our body's cells. If the traveling hormone is not the correct fit for the receptor, it continues traveling until it finds its matching puzzle piece. In this way, all the different hormones traveling throughout the body finally connect with their appropriate receptors (or intended receivers) in order to do the work for which they were produced.

The sex hormones **estrogen, progesterone,** and **testosterone,** which are produced by the ovaries and adrenal glands in women, influence us closely as females; they affect our biological functioning and our monthly cycle as well as the transitions of puberty and menopause. The thyroid hormones and the hormone **insulin,** which is produced by the **pancreas,** also affect our menstrual cycling and bodily functions.

In addition to hormones, neurotransmitters also have a huge impact on our feelings, moods, and activity level. The neurotransmitters—**endorphins, serotonin,** and **dopamine**—are brain chemicals involved in carrying messages to and from the brain. Like hormones, they tell organs and glands when and how to work. To some degree, these neurotransmitters control the functioning of our nervous system. And the fluctuations of hormones throughout the menstrual cycle directly affect and are affected by these key neurotransmitters.

Sex Hormones

Progesterone is manufactured by your adrenal glands and your ovaries. It is the primary building block for the two other sex hormones, **estrogen** and **testosterone.** Estrogen actually refers to an entire class of hormones. These are individually called **estradiol, estone,** and **estriol.** Estrogen is so important to women that your body manufactures it in several different ways. Testosterone is one of the group of hormones called **androgens.** It is considered the male sex hormone. But women normally have some testosterone too, just as men have some estrogen. Testosterone promotes major body tissue building when you're exercising.

Other Hormones: Insulin and Thyroid

The hormone **insulin,** familiar because of its role in diabetes, is secreted by the pancreas into the blood. It regulates carbohydrate metabolism by promoting the passage of glucose from the blood into the cells. In this way, insulin helps supply a constant flow of fuel for the body's cellular processes. Anything that affects insulin utilization by the body will therefore affect our body's functioning. For example, fluctuating levels of estrogen and progesterone (as experienced in perimenopause) can make us more sensitive to changes in glucose and insulin levels. Also, as we age our body becomes more insulin-resistant—with diabetes the possible result.

Iodine enters the **thyroid gland** under the influence of **TSH (thyroid stimulating hormone)** and is involved in the formation of **thyroxine (T4)** and **triiodothyronine (T3).** Thyroid hormone levels influence estrogen levels. If a person has too much thyroid hormone (**hyperthyroidism**), estrogen is metabolized more rapidly, decreasing the amount of free circulating estrogens throughout the body. Conversely, if a person has too little thyroid hormone (**hypothyroid**), she will have higher levels of circulating estrogen in her bloodstream. Abnormal thyroid function (high or low) can lead to decreased ovulation and irregular bleeding during menopause (as well as at other times). Thyroid dysfunction occurs commonly in women after menopause.

During menopause, when your body shifts naturally to lower estrogen levels, signs and symptoms of abnormal thyroid function that previously went unnoticed may become more obvious. Such signs and symptoms include rapid heartbeat, nervousness, heat intolerance, cold intolerance, heart palpitations, fatigue or weakness, weight loss, difficulty breathing, diarrhea, anorexia, and sleep disturbance. Because these are also symptoms of menopause, the proper diagnosis of abnormal thyroid function may be overlooked unless appropriate testing is performed.

Bone-mineral absorption is also tied to thyroid function. When your thyroid levels are in the normal range, bone building results. However, increased levels of thyroxine in the blood can result in bone loss. The opposite is true for estrogen. As with thyroxine, adequate estrogen in our system promotes bone building. However, when there are low levels of estrogen, more calcium leaves our bones, which will weaken them over time.

Finally, the **adrenal glands,** situated on top of the kidneys, are a major source of postmenopausal estrogen. The adrenal hormones also affect water retention and blood pressure, blood sugar levels, and other biological activity such as day and night activity cycles.

Neurotransmitters: Natural Energizers, Natural Tranquilizers

As stated earlier, there are three main types of neurotransmitters: the endorphins, serotonin, and dopamine.

Endorphins are the body's "natural opium." They affect pain perception, temperature regulation, breathing, appetite, blood pressure, learning and memory, and even sexual behavior and function.

In a woman's body, endorphin levels increase as the monthly cycle progresses and are very responsive to the fluctuating levels of estrogen and progesterone. They start out very low during the actual menstrual period, then peak just after ovulation. Unfortunately, during menopause (when we could really use them), endorphins and their desirable opiate effects are lessened since we no longer have the changing and cyclic levels of the female sex hormones. Endorphin levels, however, can be increased with exercise.

Serotonin is present in the blood, brain, and nerve tissues and is a very important mood regulator. The release of serotonin increases right before sleep. This happens for a good reason: Serotonin decreases our body's reaction to internal or external stimuli, reducing the amount of time it takes to fall asleep. It is a brain chemical that produces calm, a mood stabilizer. Because serotonin responds to the fluctuating levels of endorphins, it is sensitive to fluctuating levels of estrogen and progesterone. Unfortunately, decreased estrogen leads to decreased brain serotonin. This, in turn, may lead to abnormal sleep patterns in perimenopause and menopause, creating significant physiological and psychological changes. Falling asleep is actually less of a problem than staying asleep. This condition may be, in part, responsible for the increased incidence of depression that occurs in women during perimenopause. With our decreased serotonin and endorphin levels, we can be as sleep-deprived as a new mother who's been up all night nursing her infant!

Dopamine plays a role in body movement, motivation, primitive drives, sexual behavior, emotions, and the functioning of our immune system. Unlike serotonin, dopamine decreases at night and increases during the day. It promotes increased wakefulness, excitement, and focus. Dopamine levels are lower when estrogen levels decline. Endorphins also stimulate dopamine production. (High-protein foods are also thought to increase dopamine production.)

Clearly, estrogen strongly influences the levels of neurotransmitters in the brain. And since our thinking processes and motor activity are, in turn, managed by these neurotransmitters, changes in estrogen levels can change the way our brain cells communicate with each other and with other cells in the body. Thus, one might justifiably say that estrogen works to some extent like an intermediary helping to regulate processes throughout our entire body.

FROM MENSTRUATION TO MENOPAUSE

When we are born, we have approximately 2 million eggs in our ovaries. By the time we reach our childbearing years, this number is reduced to about 400,000. And by menopause, we have less than 30. Our supply of eggs is actually programmed to run out with the passage of time as part of the natural aging process. The ovary "raises" hundreds of follicles with hundreds of eggs each month, but only one egg is matured and expelled. In the early stages of the menstrual cycle, when the estrogen levels from the ovary begin to gradually increase, the pituitary gland responds to the hypothalamus by increasing storage and secretion of **follicle stimulating hormone (FSH)** and **luteinizing hormone (LH).** FSH and LH promote (1) the development and enlargement of the egg follicles and (2) the production of estrogen by the follicle cells. At some point, the level of estrogen reaches a critical concentration at a crucial time, which results in the significant secretion of luteinizing hormone known as the **LH surge.** Ultimately, the follicle responds to this surge by releasing a mature egg, which is propelled from the egg follicle out into the pelvic cavity and then into the fallopian tube. This process is called **ovulation.**

The remnant of the egg follicle or egg sac then becomes an endocrine gland itself. It is now called the **corpus luteum,** which is primarily responsible for producing increasing amounts of progesterone following ovulation. After ovulation, the activities of the hypothalamus and pituitary gland are suppressed by the increasing level of progesterone, which dominates the second half of the cycle. Progesterone primarily increases the thickness of the lining of the uterus (the **endometrium**) in preparation for implantation of a fertilized egg. If no fertilization has occurred, then the corpus luteum shrinks and starts to resorb, and progesterone and estrogen levels begin to decrease. The uterine lining sheds, resulting in menstrual bleeding, and the decreasing levels of hormones signal the brain to release the releasing hormones (FSH and LH). Thus, the pituitary gland is stimulated by the hypothalamus to begin the cycle again.

Perimenopause: The Changing Cycle

During perimenopause, menstruation becomes irregular or nonexistent for some, or heavy and unpredictable for others. The fewer follicles available, the less estrogen production is possible. Cycling begins to occur without actual ovulation. The function of the ovaries, which was to mature and release eggs for conception, declines and then ceases. The pituitary gland, in a desperate attempt to stimulate the ovaries, begins to release more FSH and LH in the bloodstream. Thus, levels of these pituitary hormones increase while levels of the sex hormones decrease. It is as if the brain has declared, "We are going to try to get this reproductive system jump-started with more hormones," and the ovary has responded, "No way, no more."

With no more eggs proceeding through the maturing process, there will be no more corpus luteum formation from the mature egg sac, and therefore no more progesterone. Finally, the estrogen level drops too low to stimulate the growth of the lining of the uterus. Small amounts of estrogen continue to be produced by the adrenal glands, the ovaries, and other glandular sources (such as in fatty body tissue) throughout a woman's life. However, there is not enough to make the body function as before, so menstruation stops.

In the final perimenopausal stages, we begin to experience alterations in our secondary sex characteristics and tissues. These developments are due to the significant hormonal changes described, particularly the decrease in estrogen. This transition physically affects every organ but especially the brain, the bones, and the central nervous system.

MENOPAUSE AND BEYOND

Menopause is the most common endocrine change we will experience as women in conjunction with the aging process. *However, we must not confuse the general effects of natural aging with the effects of estrogen decline and withdrawal.* It happens that aging occurs in tandem with menopause, not because of menopause. Unfortunately, we all get old! So, what can we expect from menopause? We can expect to experience varying degrees of body change and body function. (And so can men! Although it seems that men do not experience as dramatic a physiological and emotional shift as menopausal women, their production of testosterone does decline as they age.) And what can we do? We need to acknowledge the complexities and subtleties of these natural changes in order to recognize the need to overcome old and bad habits that would otherwise negatively affect our health in the future.

The Symptoms

The symptoms of menopause vary greatly from woman to woman, from no problematic signs at all to complete incapacitation by one's discomforts. Most women experience something in between these two extremes. What are the symptoms? The medical literature attributes a myriad of afflictions to menopause, starting with the oft-mentioned **hot flashes** (or **hot flushing**), which is the sudden sensation of heat in the upper body, lasting a minute or more. These can also occur at night (**night sweats**) and be followed by a pronounced chill similar to that which a fever might produce. also common are bone and joint aches, insomnia, unexplained depression or teariness, mood fluctuations, pain during intercourse (**dyspareunia**), vaginal dryness, headaches, fatigue, dizziness, strange skin sensations, forgetfulness, heart palpitations, and nightmares—just to name a few. (Some of the lists of symptoms that we have seen are even longer.) We again stress that some of these symptoms can be attributed to general aging or other health problems, so proper evaluation should always be sought.

Physical changes you may experience include the following.

1. *A decrease in the size of your reproductive system,* that is, your uterus, ovaries, and vaginal canal. You are no longer going to bear children, obviously. But this can also mean a change in your feelings of sexuality and sex-

ual comfort because of decreased vaginal lubrication and elasticity. Your local drug store has numerous products to help alleviate this condition.

2. *Some loss of muscle tone,* which is both hormonally caused and due to the natural aging process. You need to exercise to continue to promote and maintain muscular strength and flexibility, as well as continued cardiovascular health and bone strength.

3. *Normal changes in body shape,* which are also both hormonally caused and due to the natural aging process. You will look different. Your fatty tissues will be redistributed, and your metabolism will slow slightly. Some women start to look more like apples (fat in the waist) than pears (fat in the hips and thighs).

4. *Changes in the shape, firmness, and size of breast tissue.* These changes can mean less pain for the woman with a history of fibrocystic breast tissue, but may be distressing to others for aesthetic reasons.

5. *Increased hair growth (not necessarily where you want it) and skin changes.* These effects are caused by the change in the ratio of androgen-type hormones to significant estrogen hormones; they can also be inherited traits.

6. *Bone loss and changes in bone structure.* Fortunately, some of these potential bone problems can be minimized by a healthy diet and exercise regimen. Moreover, some women will choose hormone replacement therapy in part to assist in the prevention of **osteoporosis.**

The Positive Side

Women should view menopause as their special communication from nature. Think of it as a signal to actively consider choices for a healthier lifestyle. It is essential to our successful midlife rite of passage that we reevaluate our physical and emotional capabilities. We can take responsibility for the decisions that will effectively maximize our health. We have a lot of years to live following the onset of menopause, and it is important to plan our approach to those years in a way that promotes a long and healthy life. Menopause presents an opportunity for reflection, if we take the time for it. It is difficult for many of us to "find time" in our hectic lives. Time is not a gift people usually give to us, nor is it a gift we easily give ourselves. Nonetheless, making time for self-examination during menopause is something positive we can do for ourselves.

"Eliminate the negative and accentuate the positive!" Adele Davis once said. "Every day we do one of two things: We build health or produce disease in ourselves." Of course, one of the obvious things you can do to build health is to begin to evaluate your nutritional status. For what you eat is one of the most important contributors to your health—both now and in the future.

2

TO TAKE HORMONES OR NOT TO TAKE HORMONES

One of your biggest decisions as you approach menopause is whether or not to take hormones. Most hormone replacement regimens contain a combination of the hormones **estrogen** and **progestin,** which is, in either its synthetic or natural form, a version of the hormone **progesterone.** This combination treatment is referred to as **hormone replacement therapy (HRT)** and is usually given to women who still have their uterus. Another regimen, **estrogen replacement therapy (ERT),** consists solely of the hormone estrogen; it is typically given to women who have had hysterectomies. Both regimens entail both risks and benefits, and you should consider these, in light of your medical history and your doctor's recommendation, when deciding whether HRT (or ERT) is right for you.

Unfortunately, scientists don't yet have all the information any of us needs to make a fully informed decision about taking hormones. The National Institutes of Health is currently conducting a large study that will help provide more data on this question, but the results won't be available for several years. Even then, decisions will be determined by each woman's particular needs. Still, we do know some of the risks and benefits that you should consider now as you make your personal choice. We'll review each briefly.

THE BENEFITS OF HORMONE REPLACEMENT THERAPY

The well-established health benefits of HRT include protection against osteoporosis, lowered risk of heart disease, and alleviation of menopausal symptoms. The severity of menopausal symptoms, the most common being hot flashes, can vary greatly from woman to woman, but HRT appears to control many of them in most women. That sounds terrific, doesn't it? Unfortunately, HRT also involves potentially serious risks and unpleasant side effects.

17

THE RISKS AND SIDE EFFECTS OF HORMONE REPLACEMENT THERAPY

The major risk is cancer. ERT may increase your risk of endometrial cancer (in the lining of the uterus) by four times. It increases the risk of liver enlargement and tumors. Your chances of getting gallbladder disease are one-and-a-half times greater. ERT also appears to increase your risk of breast cancer if used for more than 10 years. A recent highly controversial Swedish study showed that women who took a combination of estrogen and progestin (HRT) had four times the risk of developing breast cancer compared to women who took no hormones. The doses used in this study were about twice as high as those used in the United States; nonetheless, it is still cause for concern.

The Centers for Disease Control reviewed 16 clinical studies and found that the risk of breast cancer increased with the length of estrogen replacement therapy. Harvard researchers reported in a 1991 *Consumer Reports* article that they believe estrogen may promote the growth of *existing* tumors rather than causing new ones to develop. Therefore, it makes sense for any woman considering ERT or HRT to be checked thoroughly for any tumors as part of a careful physical exam, and also to have a mammogram taken, *before* ERT or HRT is started. HRT poses particular risks if you have a history of breast or endometrial cancer, liver disease, or blood clots.

Progestin is often added to estrogen to reduce the cancer risk; however, unanswered questions remain about its true effectiveness. A recent article in *Menopause: The Journal of the North American Menopause Society* noted that combinations of estrogen and progestin may not be fully protective against endometrial cancer because cases of endometrial cancer still occur during HRT. But the article also noted that there is some preliminary evidence that adding progestin may also help protect against osteoporosis and breast cancer.

Given all this conflicting information about progestin, we definitely need more studies conducted with larger populations before any firm conclusions can be drawn. At this point, however, many researchers believe that when estrogen and progestin are used together, the risks of endometrial cancer are significantly less than when estrogen is used alone.

In addition to the cancer risks, women are also bothered by other unintended consequences, or side effects, of HRT. One recent study published in *Menopause: The Journal of the North American Menopause Society* estimated that up to 50 percent of women who were prescribed HRT stopped taking their hormones after 1 year—mainly due to unpleasant side effects. Estrogen and progestin can cause PMS symptoms, bloating, breast tenderness, headaches, nausea, and the return of menstrual bleeding. This raises the question, does HRT involve trading one set of discomforts for another? The authors of this study believed that their results were partially due to poor instructions from the health care provider. In addition, perhaps more individual adjustment of the doses would have alleviated some of the problems.

Another unfortunate (and unpopular) side effect of hormone replacement therapy is weight gain. A 1991 study done at the University of Pittsburgh followed 485 premenopausal women over 3 years. The hormone users gained an average of 7.3 pounds compared with 6.4 pounds for women with hysterectomies taking hormones and only 3.1 pounds for postmenopausal women not taking hormones. Hormone users also had the highest gains in their upper arm and hip fat fold measurements. And this side effect is more than an annoying aesthetic consideration; for as weight increases, so does the risk for many chronic ailments like heart disease and diabetes.

Finally, although it's neither a risk nor a side effect, another drawback of ERT and HRT is that their protective effects last only as long as you keep taking those estrogen pills. So it's important to know before you begin ERT or HRT that it may become a lifetime prescription—in order to continue to protect your bones and heart.

WHY SOME WOMEN SHOULD NOT TAKE HORMONES

Many women decide that the potential negatives associated with HRT outweigh the benefits for them. For some, the decision not to take hormones is made because of their medical history. Others just want to avoid the risks and side effects that go along with HRT. Still others simply prefer to live naturally, rather than adding hormones that nature did not intend.

The Harvard Women's Health Watch (1994) offers the following checklists of reasons to consider foregoing HRT.

You should absolutely not take HRT if you have:
- Current breast cancer.
- Current endometrial cancer.
- Active liver disease.
- Active thrombophlebitis or thromboembolism.
- Vaginal bleeding of unknown cause.

And although there are exceptions, you should probably not take HRT if you have:
- A history of breast cancer.
- A history of endometrial cancer.

- A history of liver disease.
- Large uterine fibroids.
- Endometriosis.
- A history of thrombophlebitis or thromboembolism.
- A history of stroke or **transient ischemic attack (TIA).**
- A history of recent heart attack.
- Pancreatic disease.
- Gallbladder disease (however, if your gallbladder has already been removed, this is no longer a problem).
- Fibrocystic breast disease (experts estimate that one in three women have fibrocystic breast tissue).
- Hypertension that is aggravated by estrogen.
- Migraine headaches aggravated by estrogen.

We further recommend that you discuss HRT carefully with your health care practitioner if you have one or more of the following conditions:

- A combination of health concerns, such as obesity, varicose veins, high blood pressure, and smoking.
- A family history of estrogen-dependent cancers (breast, uterine, and ovarian).
- Chronic unexplainable jaundice (Dublin-Johnson syndrome).
- Excess fat in the blood (hyperlipidemia) or high serum cholesterol.
- Severe hypertension (high blood pressure).
- Severe varicose veins.
- Diabetes mellitus.
- A change or increase in skin pigment formation.
- Multiple sclerosis.
- Epilepsy.
- Disorders of the immune system.
- Diseases of the kidneys.

THE CHOICE IS YOURS

Currently only about 20 percent of menopausal women in the United States opt for hormone replacement therapy, although it is prescribed more heavily in the west than in other regions. Given the risks, why is HRT such an acceptable form of menopausal therapy in some regions of the country? Perhaps because no scientifically based alternative therapies have been described in detail to the public or medical community. (However, that will probably change within the next 5 to 10 years after current studies are completed.) An additional allure of HRT is the simplicity for the woman (and her physician) of taking (or prescribing) a pill, compared to the complexity of changing her diet and lifestyle. And there is HRT's documented lowered risk of osteoporosis and heart disease. All in all, though, the advisability of HRT remains a medical dilemma.

What you have to remember is that HRT is neither good nor bad, neither right nor wrong. Your choice depends on you individually and on what your personal health needs are. Each woman will have different degrees of discomfort during menopause, and each woman will have a different risk profile for osteoporosis, heart disease, and cancer. Those women at greatest risk for osteoporosis and heart disease will reap the greatest benefits from HRT. And while there are certainly risks in taking hormones for an extended period, it's also important to put those risks in proper perspective: Other changeable and controllable conditions or lifestyle habits, such as obesity, smoking, high blood pressure, and an unhealthy diet, are considered far greater contributing factors for disease than is HRT.

Since the chief health benefits of HRT are the possible reduced risks for cardiovascular disease and osteoporosis, knowing whether you are at a high risk for either of these two diseases may help you decide whether to take hormones or not. The lists below will give you an idea where you stand on each of them.

You are at risk for cardiovascular disease (heart disease) if:
- Your total cholesterol level is over 200 mg/dL (of blood).
- Your LDL ("bad") cholesterol level is over 130 mg/dL.
- Your triglyceride count is over 200 mg/dL.
- Your HDL ("good") cholesterol is less than 35 mg/dL.
- Your ratio of serum cholesterol to HDL cholesterol is over 4.5:1 (to calculate this ratio, divide your total cholesterol count by your HDL count).
- You have high blood pressure.
- You smoke.
- You are diabetic.
- You have a family history of premature heart disease (heart disease before age 55 in one of your parents).

You are at risk for osteoporosis if:
- You are White.
- You are underweight for your height (described as skinny).
- You are fair-skinned.
- You smoke.
- Your mother or other female blood relatives grew stooped with age or had osteoporosis.

- You drink a lot of soda (carbonated beverages containing phosphoric acid).
- You take thyroid supplements.
- You have chronic digestion problems that affect how nutrients in food are absorbed.

If you have several of the risk factors for heart disease, you may want to discuss with your health care provider what steps you can take to quit smoking, lower your blood pressure, and/or improve your cholesterol counts and ratios. And if you have several of the risk factors for osteoporosis, you may want to discuss with your health care provider the benefits of taking a bone-density test to determine just how great your risk is.

HOW DIET CAN HELP IF YOU
DON'T TAKE HORMONES

Even if you decide not to take hormones during or after menopause, you can still achieve some of the benefits associated with HRT through diet alone. The chapters that follow provide specific information, but here is an overview.

You can lower your risk of osteoporosis by increasing the calcium and calcium enhancers in your diet and by decreasing the calcium depleters.

You can lower your risk of heart disease by changing your diet in several ways. You can decrease your LDL (low-density lipoprotein, or "bad") cholesterol by reducing the total amount of fat in your diet and avoiding *trans* fatty acids (created in the hydrogenation process to make margarine) and other saturated fats. You can increase your HDL (high-density lipoprotein, or "good") cholesterol by emphasizing monounsaturated fats (olive and canola oil) over saturated fats in a low-fat diet. And you can reduce your risk of blood clotting by eating more omega-3 fatty acids (found in seafood and canola oil) every day.

Dietary changes can also minimize some of the unpleasant symptoms of menopause, such as hot flashes, headaches, and so on.

HOW DIET CAN HELP IF YOU
DO TAKE HORMONES

If you *have* decided to take hormones, you can use diet to minimize the health risks and side effects associated with the treatment. For example, since HRT appears to increase the risk of some cancers, you can eat plenty of antioxidant-rich foods (antioxidants are vitamin C, vitamin E, and beta-carotene), which include cruciferous vegetables like broccoli and cauliflower, and plenty of phytochemical-rich foods, such as citrus fruits and tomatoes, all of which will help decrease your risk for cancer. (Phytochemicals are natural substances found in plants that have, among other things, cancer-fighting properties.) Following the 10 Diet Commandments described throughout the remainder of this book will also help minimize your risk of cancer and other health risks. Table 2.1 details how diet can help minimize the side effects of HRT.

Table 2.1. How Diet Can Help Minimize the Side Effects of HRT

Side Effect	Dietary Suggestions for Minimizing It
Bloating	Keep your water balance (hydration) in check by drinking at least 8 cups of water (or other decaffeinated beverages) every day, eating a fairly low-sodium diet (no more than 2,400 mg of sodium per day), and avoiding caffeine and alcohol, which are diuretics (meaning they encourage dehydration). However, "natural" diuretics (such as watermelon, lemon, grapefruit juice, and cucumber) in normal portions might help.
Breast tenderness	Work with your doctor or nurse practitioner to adjust the dose of estrogen (or use natural progesterone). In addition, some health care practitioners have observed some relief from taking 50 to 100 mg of vitamin B-6 daily and from taking evening primrose oil (very expensive, sold in pill form).
Headaches	Avoid trigger foods, which may include alcohol in red wine and beer; tyramine in aged cheeses, chianti wine, and pickled herring; chocolate; and caffeine. (It's uncertain whether chocolate causes migraines or whether chocolate cravings are actually caused by impending migraines. As for caffeine, headaches are the most common symptom of caffeine withdrawal, but if you never consume caffeine, you obviously don't have to worry about this possibility.)
Nausea	Work with your doctor or nurse practitioner to vary the dose of hormones, or the time of day the hormones are taken (evening versus morning). Also, eat small, frequent meals throughout the day, and avoid consuming stomach irritants such as coffee, spicy foods, and acidic foods (e.g., tomato and orange juice) on an empty stomach.
Weight gain	Eat a low-fat diet and plenty of fiber, fruits, and vegetables. Eat several small meals throughout the day, and eat light at night (Diet Commandment #5). Following a regular exercise program in tandem with these dietary changes will be especially effective in discouraging weight and body fat gains.

DIET IS KEY WITH OR
WITHOUT HORMONES

In summary, whether you decide to take hormones or not, your diet can help you—either by mitigating the symptoms of menopause or by minimizing the risks and side effects of HRT. And your diet can also help you reduce the risks of the diseases of aging: heart disease, cancer, and osteoporosis.

Even if you opt for HRT—either because you have a particularly high personal risk for osteoporosis or cardiovascular disease or because you have particularly debilitating menopausal symptoms—sooner or later you may decide to stop taking the hormones for good medical or personal reasons. So the sooner you start eating to improve or maintain your health, the better off you'll be.

You may be asking yourself, "Is HRT right for me? Or should I try an alternative therapy such as changing my diet?" The answer is, it isn't an either-or proposition. *Try improving your diet no matter what!*

Eating a low-fat diet, exercising regularly, maintaining your ideal weight, keeping your blood pressure low, managing your stress better, and quitting smoking now are proven ways to protect your heart against disease—and with no negative side effects. Admittedly, the drawbacks of following my 10 Diet Commandments may mean changing your diet, spending a bit more time in the kitchen, and maybe trying out a few new recipes and cooking techniques. But the benefits of making these changes outweigh the difficulties. So what do you have to lose?

If you do choose to take hormones, I recommend you follow my 10 Diet Commandments and opt for the lowest dose you can take for the shortest time you can comfortably manage.

If you choose not to take hormones, perhaps because your risks for osteoporosis and heart disease are relatively low and your menopausal symptoms relatively manageable through diet and alternative therapies, I still recommend that you follow my 10 Diet Commandments as a way to keep your menopausal symptoms in check and lower your risk of getting sick.

So either way, you're fated to follow the 10 Diet Commandments.

Part Two of the book, which begins on the following page, introduces the first five Diet Commandments. These first five Diet Commandments, which are described and explained in the next four chapters, focus on alleviating the symptoms of menopause and maintaining and improving your health through proper nutrition.

PART TWO

HOW DIET CAN MAKE YOU FEEL BETTER

3

MENU FOR A MORE COMFORTABLE MENOPAUSE

There *are* ways to address the symptoms of menopause without taking high doses of hormones. Whether or not you're taking hormones, it makes sense to:

- Eat foods that can help replicate the medical benefits of HRT (reduce the risks of heart disease and osteoporosis).
- Eat foods that can help ease the discomforts of menopause.

One of your major dietary defense tactics is to eat a diet rich in **phytoestrogens** (estrogenlike substances found in plants), getting as much natural estrogen as you can, even though these are less potent forms of estrogen. In addition, you can follow other diet therapies and take several commonsense steps to lessen or eliminate many of the specific menopausal symptoms that may be causing your distress.

Every woman experiences a different menopause, but few are comfortable throughout it. Most women have some hot flashes, and a smaller amount battle headaches and/or night sweats. Whatever your symptoms, you can adopt a dietary strategy to help lessen its impact.

DIETS FOR DISCOMFORTS

Many menopausal symptoms respond well to changes in not only what but also when you eat and drink. Menopausal discomforts aren't some inevitable curse; they're the result of hormonal changes. And the right diet can help you respond to those changes and feel better. In this chapter, I'll describe many techniques that have helped other women. You should find most, if not all, of your symptoms listed here; the corresponding dietary therapies are designed to make menopause more comfortable for you.

To many women, "comfortable menopause" probably sounds like an oxymoron. But some women definitely have a better time of it than others. Recent studies in Japan and Indonesia suggest that women in those countries have fewer menopausal symptoms, including hot flashes—possibly because their traditional diets are naturally high in phytoestrogen-rich foods. (We'll talk more about foods containing estrogen in chapter 4.)

Unless otherwise noted, all the dietary suggestions in this chapter are completely safe. In fact, some of these suggestions are dietary practices we should all be following anyway—for general health reasons—like eating light at night, eating more complex carbohydrates, and avoiding caffeine and alcohol (especially at night).

NATURAL SOLUTIONS FOR COMMON SYMPTOMS OF MENOPAUSE

If menopause hasn't hit you yet, you may want to read through the whole list of symptoms and corresponding solutions, and incorporate as many of the suggestions as you comfortably can. This may help you avoid the worst symptoms of menopause altogether. If you do start experiencing menopausal symptoms or if you already have, check this section for the suggestions regarding your specific symptoms. By eating right and also following the natural nondietary suggestions offered here, you're likely to feel fewer and milder discomforts.

Some of the dietary and herbal suggestions that follow have not been subjected to scientific scrutiny in well-designed clinical trials, so it is difficult to predict how well they will work for you. In many cases, though, these are great dietary suggestions for anyone wanting to eat healthier and feel better.

Breast Soreness

Some women experience breast soreness or pain during menopause. Some health care practitioners have observed that women tend to have more breast pain when they're under stress. So trying to lower your stress level may help relieve this symptom. But there are also two dietary approaches that may bring relief.

• *Decrease your fat consumption.* Women in one study of PMS sufferers found significant improvement on a very low-fat diet (less than 15 percent of their total daily calories from fat). My dietary recommendations actually allow a slightly higher percentage (see the discussion of Diet Commandment #8 in chapters 8 and 9).

- *Consider taking vitamin E supplements.* Clinical observations and anecdotal evidence of women's experiences suggest that you may find relief from taking vitamin E supplements of 150 to 300 IU (international units) per day (see chapter 5).

Headache

Changes in hormone levels, either because of HRT or menopause itself, may generate headaches in some women. Instead of just taking two aspirins and calling your doctor or nurse practitioner in the morning, try some of the following dietary suggestions.

- *Avoid headache trigger foods.* Between 8 and 25 percent of people with migraine headaches identify a particular food as the agent of their misery. Avoiding these **trigger foods** may be a good idea if you've been getting headaches from HRT. Three common trigger foods are:

1. Alcohol, in red wine and beer particularly.
2. Tyramine in aged cheeses, chianti wine, and pickled herring.
3. Chocolate (although here researchers are unsure whether chocolate causes the migraine or whether a craving for chocolate *is caused by* the impending headache).

- *Gradually decrease your caffeine consumption.* Regular caffeine consumption increases the body's expectation for this drug. When you give up caffeine, blood levels drop, and symptoms of caffeine withdrawal can set in—the most common of which is a headache. This is why health care providers often recommend decreasing the amount of caffeine you consume gradually.

Hot Flashes

Up to 80 percent of menopausal women have hot flashes. Fortunately, hot flashes typically subside after a year or two. Until they do, try some of the following dietary and nondietary suggestions.

- *Eat more phytoestrogen-rich foods.* Weak estrogenlike compounds found in such foods as papaya, tofu, beans, lentils, and peas are theorized to be at least partially responsible for the low incidence of hot flashes among women in Japan, where these foods are part of their traditional diet. (See also chapter 4 for further explanation and suggestions.)
- *Avoid foods that trigger hot flashes.* Caffeine, alcohol, and spicy foods trigger hot flashes in many women. When you have a hot flash, consider whether you had a triggering beverage or food earlier that day. If so, you

can try avoiding these three food categories to see whether your hot flashes lessen.

• *Avoid situations that trigger hot flashes.* Avoid emotional upsets, high temperatures, and poorly ventilated rooms. Dress in layers that can be shed as your body heat rises.

• *Consider taking ginseng.* Ginseng, the most widely used herbal remedy in the United States, has a steroidlike chemical structure, suggesting that it may have an estrogenlike effect on the body. Some health practitioners claim that moderate hot flashes can be relieved by sipping ginseng tea. However, a few reports have noted abnormal uterine bleeding with the use of ginseng, so consult your doctor if you notice anything unusual.

• *Take vitamin E supplements.* The evidence supporting vitamin E use is mostly anecdotal. However, some health practitioners claim that taking 150 to 300 IU (international units) of vitamin E a day can help relieve more moderate hot flashes. You'll have to take vitamin E supplements because getting this amount from food alone is next to impossible. There are no documented side effects to taking 300 IU of vitamin E.

• *Discuss dong quai and black cohosh herbs with your health practitioner.* These substances are not FDA-approved. Their active compounds have not been identified, and the risk and benefits of taking them are not yet clear. However, dong quai does seem to contain a natural estrogenlike substance. It may also have some therapeutic properties. At the moment, dong quai is the only herb being studied scientifically for its effects on menopausal symptoms.

Insomnia

Over-the-counter medications are probably not going to be very helpful for menopausal women with insomnia. First, try the diet and lifestyle suggestions listed here. If they don't work, then see your doctor or nurse practitioner to discuss pharmaceutical and hormonal options. These are often prescribed along with a program that encourages positive lifestyle and behavior changes.

• *Eat carbohydrates in the evening.* Sleepiness may be more likely to follow a high-carbohydrate meal than a high-protein one. (See chapter 6 for a discussion of carbohydrates and protein.) Scientists are still studying the whys and hows of this phenomenon, but some suspect the following three processes at work:

1. The amino acid **tryptophan,** found in many high-carbohydrate foods, is converted in the brain to **serotonin,** a sleep-inducing neurotransmitter.

2. A high-carbohydrate meal is thought to produce heat as a by-product of digestion and metabolism, and heat is thought to encourage sleepiness. In one study, the body's postmeal heat production peaked right around the onset of sleep.

3. High-carbohydrate meals increase the duration of total sleep by lengthening some of the individual sleep stages. Scientists are still investigating why high-carbohydrate meals have this effect.

• *Try drinking warm skim milk at bedtime.* Although it doesn't appear that a glass of milk has the chemicals to produce sleep, it may help psychologically: Warm milk reminds many of us of comforting moments when we were children.

• *Avoid stimulants like caffeine, especially after 5 P.M. or 6 P.M.* Sometimes you can solve insomnia just by eliminating caffeine from your diet, according to Gary Zammit, director of St. Luke's Sleep Disorders Institute in New York. Remember, caffeine can be found in coffee, tea, chocolate, and certain soft drinks, as well as in many prescription and over-the-counter drugs. If the after 5 or 6 rule doesn't work for you, you might want to stop consuming caffeine even earlier—say, after 1 P.M. or 2 P.M.

• *Avoid drinking alcohol late at night.* Go ahead and have your glass of wine with dinner; just abstain in the later evening hours. While alcohol may indeed help you *fall* asleep, it doesn't help you get *restful* sleep. It actually wakes you several times during the night, disturbing your deep-sleep phases, which are the most restorative. Also, it's a very bad idea to become dependent on alcohol to help you get to sleep.

• *Exercise—but wisely.* Exercise regularly, but don't exercise late in the evening. Regular exercise promotes deeper stages of sleep, especially exercising in the late afternoon or early morning. Exercising at 6 P.M. or 7 P.M. is probably fine if you're retiring at 10 P.M. or 11 P.M.

• *Don't go to bed really hungry.* Hunger, if it's strong enough, can wake you up, thereby shortening your sleep. Before going to bed, you may want to try having a carbohydrate snack (fruit, bread, or low-fat crackers), but not one high in protein.

Moodiness/Sadness

Some menopausal women experience mood swings and periods of sadness similar to the emotional surges many women describe as PMS. Mood changes may be due, in part, to lack of sleep, so see the suggestions listed under "Insomnia," "Hot Flashes," and "Night Sweats." It may also help to avoid certain dietary substances, as described below.

- *Avoid alcohol,* which is generally considered to be a depressant.
- *Avoid caffeine,* which is a stimulant that results, for many people, in a high-energy/low-energy, up-and-down response.
- *Avoid eating concentrated sweets on an empty stomach.* For some people, eating sweets on an empty stomach results in a short-lived high-energy response, which is then followed by an insulin spurt and the resultant low blood sugar. Low blood sugar can make some people feel sluggish and moody.

Night Sweats

Twenty-five to 40 percent of menopausal women have night-sweating episodes. Keep your bedroom temperature cool at night, and also follow the suggestions listed under "Hot Flashes."

Urinary-Tract Infections

Declining estrogen levels cause the tissues lining the bladder to become thinner, making it easier for bladder infections (urinary-tract infections) to develop. To ward off such infections, try the following dietary and behavioral changes.

- *Drink lots of liquids.* Drink plenty of noncaffeinated beverages and water. Drinking lots of liquids keeps the bladder full and flushing frequently, so the level of bacteria in the bladder is diluted. However, avoid caffeinated and alcoholic beverages, which are diuretics (meaning that they stimulate your kidneys to release water into the bladder), and so are more likely to encourage dehydration.
- *Urinate frequently.* Remember to urinate frequently, especially following sex. Again, flushing out your system prevents bacterial concentration.
- *Drink cranberry juice.* A 6-month study of postmenopausal elderly women showed that drinking 10 ounces of cranberry juice a day lowered the amount of bacteria and white blood cells in urine. Researachers theorize that a substance in cranberry juice keeps the problem bacteria from clinging to the wall of the urinary tract, where they can multiply and cause infection and painful urination. Low-calorie cranberry juice beverages, containing only 50 calories a cup, are available in most supermarkets.

Vaginal Atrophy

When estrogen levels drop, the tissue lining the vagina becomes thinner, and normal vaginal secretions decline. Intercourse can become painful. About 50 percent of menopausal women experience changes in their vaginal tissue. To minimize or counteract these changes, try the following nondietary solutions.

- *Consider using estrogen creams.*   Estrogen cream, when applied regularly, can restore the vaginal mucosa. But be aware that estrogen can be absorbed into the bloodstream this way. Thus, if you have decided to avoid taking estrogen supplements, you may want to avoid using the cream, too. However, the level of estrogen that you will take in from estrogen cream will certainly be much lower than from HRT.
- *Use vaginal moisturizers and lubricants.*   There are several water-based vaginal moisturizers and lubricants, such as Astroglide, available in your pharmacy that are often effective. Your mucous membranes are themselves water-based and therefore an oil-based lubricant such as Vaseline is more likely to adhere and cause irritation.
- *Have sex regularly.*   That's right! Sex in and of itself can help preserve your vaginal walls, perhaps by increasing blood flow to the area. In one study, postmenopausal women who had sex more than three times a week had less vaginal atrophy than those who had sex less than ten times a year. And here's a bonus: Sex also helps make your vaginal area more acidic, which helps protect against infection.

You'll notice as you read the rest of this book that many of the dietary suggestions mentioned above are incorporated into the 10 Diet Commandments. Which of these dietary suggestions are of particular significance to you, of course, depends on your personal symptoms and your body's response. Try the dietary suggestions described above for the particular symptoms you're experiencing, but then try following all 10 Diet Commandments. They are important not only during menopause but for all your postmenopausal years as well.

4

UPPING YOUR ESTROGEN NATURALLY

Estrogen is one of those hormones most women never really think about before menopause, except maybe if they contemplate using birth control pills. Then menopause hits, hot flashes and all, and suddenly estrogen, or the lack of it, is *all* we can think about.

As explained in chapter 1, during menopause your ovaries produce less and less estrogen. This sudden lack of estrogen is what causes many of the discomforts of menopause. It is also what dramatically raises the risks of heart disease and osteoporosis for postmenopausal women, because estrogen, to some degree, protects women from accelerated bone loss and several heart disease risk factors.

For years women have thought that the only way to raise their estrogen level again was to take a pill. As explained in chapter 2, hormone replacement therapy (or estrogen replacement therapy) is currently the established way of temporarily restoring estrogen levels. However, if you'd rather not embark on your menopausal journey with estrogen pills at your bedside, or if you are not a candidate for HRT due to one or more of the risk factors detailed earlier, you face a very important question: "Can I increase my estrogen naturally?"

We don't yet know the complete answer to that question, but preliminary research does allow us to make some exciting and encouraging common-sense suggestions. So far, it seems, there are two ways to eat your way to higher estrogen levels during menopause and beyond: You can eat plant foods that contain weak forms of estrogen (phytoestrogens), and you can eat foods that are rich in **boron,** a mineral, abundant in plant foods, that appears to double estrogen levels in menopausal women.

The first part of this chapter will provide information on phytoestrogens, while the latter part will provide information on boron.

THE POWER OF ESTROGEN-RICH FOODS

How about raising your estrogen level by eating a bushel of broccoli, a handful of dates, or a tub of tofu? The good news is that preliminary research indicates you can actually eat your way to higher estrogen levels with a little help from some of your plant friends. For all of the estrogenlike dietary substances discovered so far come from plant foods: fruits, vegetables, legumes, and seeds—in short, natural sources. The better news is that these are foods we should all be eating more of for other health reasons anyway.

So far, scientists have identified at least 300 plants with estrogenlike components—common plants like carrots, corn, apples, barley, and oats. Further, soybeans, and soybean-based products such as tofu, are thought to be particularly potent estrogen enhancers—meaning that they enhance the level of estrogen already being produced in your body.

How the Right Diet Can Increase Your Estrogen Level

The way certain foods or nutrients seem to influence estrogen levels in the body is quite complicated. Much of the information we have on this comes from research studying the effects of substances in food on estrogen-dependent cancers, such as breast and uterine cancer, rather than on menopausal symptoms.

A few years ago, scientists began to observe that compounds in many plant foods we eat have a structure similar to the hormone estrogen that women's bodies normally produce. These **phytoestrogens** (from the Greek *phyto,* meaning "plant") can either block or enhance estrogen action in the body, depending on whether you are pre-, peri-, or postmenopausal. When you are premenopausal and your estrogen levels are high, the phytoestrogens attach to estrogen receptors, thereby inactivating some of the potent estrogens circulating in your body. This action is beneficial because it decreases the risk that you will develop estrogen-dependent cancers. On the other hand, when you are perimenopausal (undergoing menopause) or postmenopausal, when your potent estrogen levels are low or almost nonexistent, phytoestrogens act like a weaker version of estrogen. This mimicry helps protect the body from menopausal symptoms and diseases such as heart disease and osteoporosis. In either case, the overall effect of phytoestrogens on your body's health is positive.

Why You Should Use Diet to Boost Your Estrogen Level

If you have concluded that HRT just isn't right for you, then you may be looking for safe, alternative ways to boost your estrogen level during and after menopause. A phytoestrogen-rich diet may be just what you're looking

for. And even if you have chosen HRT, supplementing the hormone replacement therapy with a diet rich in phytoestrogens may enable you to take the
lowest dose possible and still find relief from many of the symptoms of
menopause. Moreover, weak estrogens in the diet may provide postmenopausal women with some of the protection from heart disease and osteoporosis that their natural estrogen did before menopause.

What about the risk of developing estrogen-dependent cancers? All of
the food sources of phytoestrogens are plant-based—which means that most
of them also contain scores of compounds that are believed to help prevent
cancer, such as indoles, beta-carotene, fiber, and vitamin C. Thus, they protect you from cancer at the same time that they address your menopausal
symptoms. (For more about disease prevention, see chapter 8.)

Evidence That a Phytoestrogen-Rich Diet Relieves Menopausal Symptoms

Very few studies have been done on the relationship between diet and menopausal symptoms. But the few that do exist are very encouraging. In one
study, dietary therapies brought relief quickly. The diets of 25 postmenopausal women were supplemented with soy flour and linseed (both of
which are high in phytoestrogens). After only 2 weeks, the women showed
significantly increased vaginal cell maturation (a measure of estrogen activity), which could bring relief from vaginal dryness, a common peri- and
postmenopausal symptom. The results of studies on larger groups of women
have also been positive.

Learning from Women in Other Cultures

It's always a good idea to examine cultures in which people already eat the
kind of diet being proposed. Who currently eats foods that are high in phytoestrogens? Who eats ample tofu and other soybean products and legumes
by the bushelful? Who makes it a habit to have plenty of fruits and vegetables, including cruciferous vegetables (a strong-tasting family that includes
bok choy, cabbage, cauliflower, kale, Brussels sprouts, turnips, and broccoli), which are particularly high in phytoestrogens? The answer: Many
Asians do.

Recent research shows that Japanese women who ate traditional, low-
fat, plant-based diets with lots of tofu (in other words, a high-phytoestrogen
diet) reported fewer hot flashes during menopause. These women also had
significantly lower rates of breast cancer. But how do we know that these
differences are related to estrogen levels? The answer is in the urine.

Because phytoestrogens compete with human estrogen in the body, one
way researchers study the effect of diet on estrogen levels in women is to
measure the amount of estrogen excreted in their urine (not a very glamorous

study technique, but very informative). Researchers have found repeatedly that, no matter which population groups they study, women eating diets high in plant foods excrete significantly more estrogen in their urine. One study showed that Japanese women eating traditional diets had significantly higher levels of estrogen in their urine compared with American and Finnish women. Another study showed that women who did not eat meat or dairy products had higher levels of estrogen in their urine than women who did.

Learning from Vegetarians

Vegetarian diets, like traditional Asian diets, tend to rely more heavily on plant-based foods than do the diets of omnivores (people who eat meat—and everything else). But American vegetarians may or may not be eating an abundance of tofu or cruciferous vegetables, and may or may not be eating a low-fat diet, habits entrenched in Asian culture and cuisine. Still, comparative studies could be revealing.

In fact, not much research has been done on the estrogen levels of peri- or postmenopausal vegetarians. However, one study did show that young vegetarian women in the United States tend to have lower estrogen levels than nonvegetarian women. These results support the idea that plant estrogens attach to estrogen receptors, thus displacing the normal potent estrogens produced in the body. And where do these displaced potent estrogens go? The body excretes them in the urine and feces.

Be Wary of Foods That Decrease Your Estrogen Level

Not surprisingly, while some foods can increase your estrogen level during and after menopause, other foods can contribute to lowering estrogen levels in those periods. The two substances implicated so far, to even a minor degree, are caffeine and, surprisingly, a diet high in one type of fiber, wheat bran.

Caffeine and Estrogen

Caffeine, found in coffee, tea, cola drinks, and many other popular beverages, has already been suspected of having certain negative effects on health if consumed in large amounts. Now there may be another reason to moderate your consumption. A study in the *American Journal of Clinical Nutrition* found that as caffeine intake went up, the amount of one type of serum estrogen (free estradiol) went down. On that evidence alone, it's probably best to at least limit your caffeine consumption during menopause as much as you can.

High Fiber and Estrogen

Many scientists now believe that fiber may play a protective role against certain cancers by increasing the breakdown of estrogen and increasing the amount of estrogen eliminated from the body through waste. The fiber seems to bind to the estrogens present in the intestines and carry them out of the body. So wouldn't fiber be disastrous to the menopausal or postmenopausal woman working to increase her estrogen level? Not necessarily.

We still know very little about the relationship between fiber and estrogen. For example, one recent study found that serum estrogen levels were *not* affected when premenopausal women's diets were supplemented with oat bran or corn bran. The women's estrogen levels did decrease, however, when their diets were supplemented with wheat bran.

So, should you stop eating whole-wheat bread and wheat-bran cereals? Of course not. Constipation plagues many women over 50, and fiber is the best way to avoid it. But try to consume a variety of different fiber types, without overreliance on wheat bran. Your body needs different types of fiber for different reasons. The fiber from oats and legumes (soluble fiber that dissolves or swells in water), for example, helps improve your blood lipid levels. While the fiber found in wheat bran and many vegetables (which is insoluble) helps food waste move quickly through the intestines, helping reduce constipation and the risk for some types of cancer.

Do We Know Enough to Act?

There are still some unanswered questions about phytoestrogens. Will weak estrogens in food *significantly* reduce the common symptoms and discomforts of menopause? Do women consuming a phytoestrogen-rich diet suffer from fewer postmenopausal chronic diseases? Conclusive research still needs to be done. But we can't wait for the complete answers to these questions before starting to act wisely by eating wisely now.

There have been few studies on the effects of diet on menopausal symptoms, and there are unlikely to be any on this topic soon, because of too few research dollars and other research priorities. Nor is private industry likely to spend a great deal of time and money studying the medicinal powers of foods, since the results probably wouldn't give them a product to sell. Still, the scientific evidence we have thus far indicates that phytoestrogens do relieve some of the symptoms of menopause and do reduce the risks of certain diseases prevalent in postmenopausal women, even though these effects haven't been clinically tested in humans to any great extent. In the best of all worlds, we could study a group of women eating a phytoestrogen-rich diet over a period of time to see whether they indeed had fewer menopausal discomforts. But most interested researchers believe that this type of study would probably never be funded. So, what do you do in the meantime? Your menopausal clock is ticking.

Fortunately, all the dietary suggestions intended to increase your estrogen naturally offer many other health rewards apart from relieving menopausal symptoms and other estrogen-related benefits. That is, they add more fiber, antioxidants, and other vitamins and minerals to your diet, while contributing little fat and no cholesterol.

HOW TO UP YOUR ESTROGEN NATURALLY

Upping your estrogen naturally entails two dietary acts: (1) eating more phytoestrogen-rich foods, and (2) eating more boron-rich foods, which appear to increase serum estrogen levels. To do so, you don't have to turn vegetarian; you just have to eat certain plant foods that are particularly rich in boron and/or phytoestrogens. Fortunately, this strategy is neither as unappetizing nor as difficult as it might at first sound. Many of these highly desirable plant foods are available in most supermarkets and easy to prepare—and most are already commonly consumed and enjoyed.

Eat Phytoestrogen-Rich Foods

Thus we arrive at the first Diet Commandment:

DIET COMMANDMENT #1

Eat at Least One Phytoestrogen-Rich Food Every Day

The two main kinds of phytoestrogens are **lignans** and **isoflavonoids.** When acted on by bacteria in the digestive tract, lignans are converted into compounds that are structurally similar to estrogen. Isoflavonoids, on the other hand, act as weak estrogen when estrogen is *not* being produced by the body during and after menopause. Before menopause, though, isoflavonoids seem to act as *anti*estrogens by inhibiting estrogen synthesis and by binding to estrogen receptors. Lignans and isoflavonoids are mostly found in different kinds of plant-based foods.

Where to Get Lignans

Your body forms lignans from fibrous components in such foods as seeds, especially flaxseed, and, to a lesser extent, in some fruits and vegetables, cereals, and legumes. Recently, researchers were able to mimic the body's production of lignans to measure the amount of lignans produced when certain foods are eaten. So we now know the best food sources of lignans. These are listed in Table A.1 in appendix A.

One of the most significant sources of lignans, but one little-known to the public, is flaxseed. Flaxseed consumption has been shown to lengthen the luteal phase of the menstrual cycle, by 1 to 2 days. This, along with other indirect evidence, suggests that these lignans, which are produced by intestinal bacteria, may act as hormonelike substances. In addition, consuming this fibrous seed could have other health benefits also. For instance, two studies done so far have shown that flaxseed seems to be a powerful anticholesterol agent, attacking the LDL, or "bad," cholesterol.

A word of warning, though: If you are considering adding flaxseed to your diet, start slowly. Some people have an allergic reaction to flaxseed, and it can cause flatulence and bloating in people not accustomed to eating it. However, once your body is used to the food, you may tolerate it better.

Where to Get Isoflavonoids

You'll find many sources of isoflavonoids in the produce department of your local supermarket. Certain fruits, vegetables, and legumes are known to be good sources. And please note that you'll get two phytoestrogens for the price of one when you buy soybeans or tofu, because soy products are considered to be sources of both isoflavonoids and lignans. Foods rich in isoflavonoids are listed in Table A.2 in appendix A.

Boost Your Boron Consumption

We now come to the second Diet Commandment.

DIET COMMANDMENT #2

Eat at Least One Boron-Rich Food Every Day

Boron is a mineral. Studies from the USDA's Human Nutrition Laboratory showed that a high-boron diet (3 mg per day) doubled the level of circulating serum estrogen in postmenopausal women and also decreased the amount of calcium being excreted by 40 percent. Though some foods high in boron also contain phytoestrogens, that's not their only estrogen-enhancing benefit. The boron itself seems to increase the body's ability to hold on to estrogen that becomes available. So it's a good idea to add some of these foods to your daily diet. See Table 4.1 for a list of foods rich in boron.

Generally speaking, fruits, vegetables, tubers, and legumes have much higher concentrations of boron than cereals, grains, and animal products. So, where would you go if you wanted to boost your boron consumption a bit?

Table 4.1.   Top Food Sources of Boron*

Food Source	Boron Content**	Food Source	Boron Content**
Plum (prune when dried)	25.5	Spinach	4.0
Quince	16.0	Carrot	3.6
Strawberry	16.0	Grapefruit	3.3
Peach	15.0	Rutabaga (root)	3.0
Cabbage	14.5	Butter bean	3.0
Dandelion (leaf)	12.5	Orange	2.8
Apple	11.0	Rutabaga (stem)	2.4
Asparagus	10.4	Endive	2.4
Celery (root)	10.3	Pea (seed)	2.3
Fig	10.0	Broccoli (stem)	2.1
Tomato	9.6	Brussels sprouts (stem)	2.1
Lettuce	8.7	Chinese cabbage	2.1
Broccoli (leaf)	8.5	Turnip (root)	2.0
Pear	8.2	Chicory (root)	2.0
Beet	8.0	Sweet potato	2.0
Sour cherry	8.0	Cauliflower (stem)	1.8
Red currant	8.0	Bell pepper	1.8
Cauliflower (floret)	7.6	Soybean	1.8
Apricot	7.0	Banana	1.8
Radish	6.4	Mango	1.8
Black currant	6.4	Cantaloupe	1.7
Celery (seed)	6.1	Wheat (seed)	1.6
Brussels sprouts (leaf)	5.7	Papaya	1.5
Cowpeas	5.7	Gooseberry	1.5
Rutabaga (leaf)	5.2	Corn	1.5
American persimmon	5.0	Mandarin orange	1.4
Grape	5.0	Avocado	1.3
Cucumber	4.6	Red raspberry	1.3
Onion	4.5	Sesame seed	1.3
Alfalfa	4.5	Blueberry	1.3
Black bean (fruit and seed)	4.5		

*Several different laboratories have released tables listing the boron content of particular foods. These tables may indicate slightly different amounts because it is difficult to measure the exact boron content of foods.

**mg per 100 g of dried food

(*continued next page*)

Table 4.1. (continued)

Food Source	Boron Content**	Food Source	Boron Content**
Spices and Herbs			
American ginseng	9.6	Sage	4.1
Opium poppy (seed)	9.5	Clove	4.0
Parsley	5.4	Rosemary	3.9
Cumin	5.0	Summer savory	3.7
Marjoram	4.8	Winter savory	3.6
Black cherry (leaf)	4.8	Fennel	3.6
Common thyme	4.6	European nettle	3.6
Evening primrose	4.1	Basil	3.1
Wild oregano	4.1	Coriander	2.9

*mg per 100 g of dried food

Source: James A. Duke, Economic Botanist, USDA Agricultural Research Service.

The produce section of your supermarket. And since boron is a mineral, when fruit is dried, the boron content remains the same per piece of fruit; but per ounce or per cup, the amount of boron goes up. So many of the best sources of boron are dried fruits like dried apples or peaches and prunes.

5

GOOD NUTRITION CAN KEEP YOU YOUNG

Menopause marks a monumental change in every woman's life, a time when we probably think about our age and future years more than ever before. This chapter gives an overview of age-related complications and how you can eat to minimize them. Some of the major issues fo aging for women, such as osteoporosis, heart disease, and cancer, are simply introduced here, and covered in greater detail in subsequent chapters.

What you eat today is an investment for tomorrow. Most people, if given the choice, want to live longer. And if they do live longer, they want to feel great and enjoy that longer life. It's an unfortunate fact of life that aging is associated with declining bodily functions. The good news is, we know that this deterioration takes place at different rates in different people. While genetic factors play a part, could the people with a slower rate of aging be doing something right? The answer is yes, because a healthy diet and lifestyle can slow many aspects of the natural aging process.

Many people, including scores of prospective investors, are waiting for mythical or scientific discoveries that will prolong life and youth. But all of us already hold the secret to prolonging life: It lies in knowing how not to shorten it. And that's about as close as we're going to get to the proverbial fountain of youth.

We can keep our bodies, skin, and organs young by avoiding substances and activities that promote aging, cause disease, or damage cells. By now we are all aware of three basic rules:

1. Don't smoke (smoking speeds bone and lung deterioration, and may lead to heart disease and a variety of cancers).
2. Don't drink too much (excessive alcohol consumption disturbs normal metabolism).
3. Avoid overexposure to the sun, and use sunscreen (ultraviolet radiation enhances skin aging and may cause skin cancer).

And there are many more ways to slow the effects of aging on your body. This chapter describes what you can do to help yourself.

HOW MAJOR ORGANS AGE AND WHAT YOU CAN DO ABOUT IT

Some of us would rather not know how many brains cells we're losing or what life is like as a 55 year old kidney, but if you know how your organs deteriorate with age, you can better understand how to slow down this process when possible.

Keep Your Heart Young

As we get older, cells of the heart muscle die and are replaced by fat and connective tissue. The heart then loses some of its contractile strength and ability to relax. The capacity of the heart to speed up during exercise (maximum heart rate) decreases in our later years. The heart loses about 1 percent of its reserve pumping capacity each year after age 30, which means with every contraction (or heartbeat) the heart is delivering less freshly oxygenated blood to body tissues.

Over the years, fatty substances in your bloodstream collect on the inner walls of arteries. These substances eventually harden, and the arterial passageway for the blood becomes narrower (atherosclerosis,) making it more difficult for the heart to pump the blood through and putting additional strain on the aging heart. The blood vessel walls also thicken with collagen deposits and lose their ability to dilate and contract in response to the heart's pumping action. So it's no surprise that blood pressure tends to increase with age.

But there is hope for a healthier heart. Some degree of **atherosclerosis** (fatty deposits on the insides of arterial walls) is an expected result of aging, but you can modulate this process by your dietary and lifestyle choices. For instance, eating a diet that is low in fat, saturated fat, and cholesterol reduces arterial clogging. (See chapter 8 for details.) Further, some cardiac researchers, including Dr. Harvey Simon at Harvard Medical School, claim there is enough evidence to blame much of the negative changes observed in the hearts of elderly people on disease and disuse rather than natural aging. If so, we would all benefit from an exercise program that properly conditions the heart and lungs.

Save Your Skeletal System

Your skeletal system, no matter what age, is in a constant state of tearing down and rebuilding. One type of bone cell is taking old bone away at the same time that another type of bone cell is replacing it with new bone.

Around the age of 30, you begin to lose more bone than you rebuild. This process begins slowly but really kicks into high gear following menopause, due to a reduction in estrogen levels.

Here are some steps you can take to discourage the loss of skeletal bone mass (see also chapter 7 for more details):

- Maximize your intake of calcium and calcium enhancers—substances that enhance how well the body absorbs and holds onto calcium (lactose, vitamin D, and magnesium).
- Minimize your intake of calcium depleters—substances that help decrease absorption or deplete the body of calcium via urine, such as excessive phosphorus (contained in soft drinks), caffeine, protein, and alcohol.
- Do weight-bearing aerobic exercise several times a week (exercise such as walking or running that requires the major bones of your body to support your entire weight).

Maintain Your Muscle Mass

Muscle mass and muscle strength also tend to decline with advancing age, because you start losing more and more muscle fibers and the nerves that help stimulate them. But you enhance your muscle mass through strength training and regular exercise. (For more information on strength training, see chapter 6.) In terms of diet, you should make sure you are getting enough protein (about 15 percent of your calories from protein) because we need sufficient protein in our diets to help maintain muscle mass. But don't eat too much protein. Excess protein doesn't build or strengthen muscle; excess protein that isn't needed for current energy is usually just converted to fat for storage. The only way to build muscle is to use muscle.

Keep Your Digestive System Dapper

Aging changes the digestive system in several ways. We can minimize some of these changes through diet. However, others require us to adjust because they affect our dietary needs.

As with many muscles in the body, the strength and elasticity of the gastrointestinal tract walls (from the mouth to the rectum) diminish with age. There are fewer contractions to help move food through. This means that constipation can become a much more common concern. Eating a diet high in fiber helps compensate for this, along with drinking more liquids.

When you reach middle age, the body makes fewer of some digestive enzymes. As a result, nutrients like calcium, vitamin B-12, zinc, and ferric iron may not be absorbed at the same rate as before. In order to keep healthy, therefore, you'll need to take in more of those vitamins and minerals. And the assorted organs that assist in digestion, such as the gallbladder, pancreas, and liver, also become more sluggish. The gallbladder releases a bit less bile into the small intestine, the pancreas produces less of the enzyme that helps break down food fat in the intestines, and the liver needs more time to metabolize drugs and alcohol because it's smaller and receives less blood.

Here are some easy-to-follow suggestions on how to keep your digestive system functioning comfortably and how to allow your body to get the most complete nutrition possible from what you eat:

- Eat smaller, more frequent meals.
- Eat a diet low in fat.
- Eat a diet rich in fiber.
- Eat more fruits and vegetables.
- Limit your consumption of alcohol.

Improve Your Immune System

The effectiveness of your immune system also declines with age. **Natural killer cells** (a component of your immune defense system) start their decline as early as your twenties. And a gland that is very important to the immune system, the **thymus** (a small gland in the neck responsible for teaching a type of white blood cell, T cells, how to coordinate the body's defense system) begins to shrink shortly after puberty, then gradually degenerates until it disappears in old age. As the thymus shrinks, fewer fighting T cells remain. Other major immune soldiers, **B lymphocytes** (another type of white blood cell), also lose with age their abilities to combat invaders such as viruses and bacteria and to release antibodies. In addition, studies show that as we age, substances known as **free radicals** can accumulate in the body, weakening our immune system and making us more vulnerable to infections and disease.

Laboratory studies have also found that certain **carotenoids**, found in certain vegetables, and vitamin E boost the activity of the disease-fighting white blood cells. **Antioxidants** (primarily vitamin C and beta-carotene) found in many fruits and vegetables seem to be able to help neutralize these worrisome free radicals. Getting enough antioxidants (beta-carotene and other carotenoids, vitamin E, and vitamin C) can help combat these immune deficiencies. But unfortunately, the elderly are less likely than other adults to eat enough of several vitamins and minerals known to help the immune response. Studies seem to indicate that supplementing your diet with certain nutrients at levels slightly more than the recommended daily amounts can improve certain measures of immune response. In one recent study researchers provided participants with 500 extra calories from food and a food supplement that supplied at least the RDA of selected vitamins and minerals. In just 8 weeks, many measures of immune response improved.

Some of the nutrients suggested as having some positive effects on the immune system are:

- Antioxidants in general and vitamins E, C, and beta-carotene and other carotenoids specifically.
- Vitamin B-6.
- Folic acid.
- Zinc.
- Adequate protein.

While definitive studies have yet to be done, eating foods that contain these nutrients certainly isn't going to hurt you—and it seems likely that it will help.

Keep Your Kidneys Young

As you age, your body sends increasingly less blood to nourish your kidneys. The kidneys also gradually lose their filtering units known as nephrons. These changes make it more and more difficult for the kidneys to do their vital job of extracting waste from the blood and concentrating it into urine. The kidneys begin to need more time and more water in order to remove the same amount of waste as they did when you were younger. So your drinking habits become very important. This would be fine if your bladder were cooperating. But, alas, bladder capacity also declines with age. So if you're treating your kidneys right by drinking plenty of fluids, you may be visiting the restroom more often. To help keep your kidneys young, try these commonsense suggestions:

- Drink plenty of water (8 cups daily is the goal) and other noncaffeinated drinks such as juice to keep your urine diluted and the kidneys well flushed.
- Limit your consumption of caffeinated beverages (caffeine is a diuretic; it forces your kidneys to get rid of more water than it should, encouraging dehydration).
- Limit your intake of alcoholic beverages (alcohol is also a diuretic).

I mentioned limiting your intake of caffeine and alcohol earlier as ways to save your skeletal system. There are also many other reasons to drink plenty of water, besides benefiting your kidneys. Your body uses water (as a component of body fluids) to transport substances around the body; to serve as lubricants and cushions in body joints, the digestive tract, and other body tissues; and to keep the body's core temperature stable. But women during menopause and after can't rely solely on thirst as an indicator of their water needs. For as we grow older, our sense of thirst has a tendency to weaken. Therefore, taking in the right amount of the right kind of fluids becomes important enough to be one of the Diet Commandments.

DIET COMMANDMENT #3

Limit Your Intake of Caffeine, Soft Drinks, and Alcohol—
and Drink Plenty of Water

See chapter 7 for more information on the effects of caffeine and alcohol, and chapters 9 and 10 for tips on modifying your drinking habits.

Strengthen Your Senses

You may not notice how your senses weaken as you age because these changes happen slowly. But that doesn't make them any less important.

Taste
Your sense of taste weakens as your taste buds age, making herbs and spices even more valuable. Smoking also dulls your taste buds, so abstaining from smoking, along with other health benefits of quitting, can help you maintain your ability to enjoy food.

Sight
Get your eyes checked regularly, whether you currently wear glasses or not, because natural aging of the proteins in the lens of the eye can lead to cataracts and other eye abnormalities. Also, make sure you're eating your carrots and other food sources of vitamin A and beta-carotene, to help your night-eyesight remain at its best.

HOW AGING CHANGES YOUR BODY SHAPE AND COMPOSITION

The changes your body shape and composition are likely to go through as you age may at first appear particularly disconcerting. But knowledge is power: If you know what changes to expect, you can act to minimize them.

Your Body Composition

The body is composed primarily of water, bone, protein (muscle mass), and fat. As you age, three of these four tend to decrease: total body water, bone density, and muscle mass. That leaves one that tends to increase—fat. By exercising regularly (including some type of strength training and weight-bearing aerobic exercise) and following the 10 Diet Commandments, you'll help minimize the bone and muscle losses while also minimizing any fat gains. And you can keep your hydration in balance by drinking lots of water and avoiding diuretic beverages such as caffeine and alcohol.

Your Body Shape

In terms of body shape, time deals us all a double whammy: Not only do postmenopausal women have on average 20 percent more fat mass than premenopausal women, but this new excess fat usually becomes distributed above the waist rather than on the hips, buttocks, and thighs. And unfortunately, this tendency toward an apple shape, as opposed to the more typical premenopausal pear shape, is associated with an increased risk of heart disease (more weight around the middle puts more strain on the heart). Perhaps because of the drop in estrogen levels, postmenopausal women's risk of heart disease starts to resemble that of a man's—just as their torso tends toward the man's classic pot-bellied apple shape as well.

THE 10 MOST-WANTED NUTRIENTS

As women get older, do they need to take in more or fewer essential nutrients? In general, the answer is more. For there are three main ways that aging affects your need for vitamins and minerals:

1. Research suggests that some of the effects of aging can be discouraged by the action of certain vitamins and minerals.
2. As we age, it can become more difficult for the body to digest, absorb, and use the vitamins and minerals it needs to function optimally.
3. Our reserve and storage capacity for vitamins and minerals also diminishes with age.

These three factors increase your need for many (though not all) essential vitamins and minerals. While extra nutrients can help, however, you also need to be careful not to overconsume vitamins and minerals through supplements as you age, because your clearance system (the kidneys) and your metabolic breakdown and detoxification system (the liver) experience some deterioration as well—and thus have a harder time processing and disposing of any excess nutrients.

Despite these important changes in nutrient needs, the government, which is responsible for setting and revising the RDAs (Recommended Daily Allowances), has not yet established a different set of RDAs for women over 50. However, based on some research and the opinions of several leading experts, it's time for them to make some. Which brings us to the fourth Diet Commandment.

DIET COMMANDMENT #4

Get about 150 Percent of the RDA for the Vitamins and
Minerals You Need More of As You Age

Vitamins and Minerals for Menopause and Beyond

The Alliance for Aging Research, a Washington, DC–based health advocacy group, now advises older Americans to take at least 250 milligrams (mg) of vitamin C, 100 international units (IU) of vitamin E, and 17,000 IU of beta-carotene daily, in order to ward off chronic diseases. As long as you like fruits and vegetables, you should be able to get this higher level of vitamin C and beta-carotene without taking supplements; however, the most vitamin E you can get from food sources is about 25 IU.

The Alliance's advice is based on recommendations from a panel consisting of researchers who already believe in the beneficial effects of antioxidant supplements. This panel reviewed more than 200 studies on antioxidants conducted over the last 20 years. However, the majority of scientific researchers contend that we still don't have enough evidence to make this recommendation. Given the preliminary evidence, it makes sense to try to consume two to three times the RDA for vitamin C (which would be 120 to 180 mg) and beta-carotene (the RDA for beta-carotene is included in the total RDA given for vitamin A), especially since it is easy to do this by eating common fruits and vegetables. Getting more vitamin E, however, especially as much as 100 IU, requires taking a supplement. Is there enough evidence to support this? The scientific jury is definitely still out on this issue. I myself take 400 IU of vitamin E daily. However, you may want to discuss your needs in this area with your doctor.

What follows now are descriptions of the vitamins some experts think women need more of as they age. The antioxidants (vitamin C, vitamin E, and beta-carotene) are listed first, followed by the remaining three vitamins and four minerals in alphabetical order. (See also Diet Commandment #7, regarding antioxidants, which is presented in chapter 8.)

Vitamin C
What does vitamin C do?
- It helps maintain and repair connective tissue (which binds the body's cells together), such as the skin or the tissue around bones and teeth.
- It keeps capillaries and other blood vessels strong.

- It helps synthesize stress hormones and thyroxin, which regulate metabolism.
- It assists in fighting off germs and disease.

How much do women over 50 need?
The current RDA for vitamin C is 60 milligrams for adult women of all ages. The Alliance for Aging Research, however, advises Americans to take larger amounts (250 mg). About 120 to 180 milligrams a day is probably a good goal for now, given what we currently know.

Why might older women need more than the RDA?
Higher intakes of vitamin C from food have been associated with a reduced risk of heart disease, some cancers, and cataracts. And there is some evidence that the antioxidant group, of which vitamin C is a member, may help slow the aging process.

Where do we get it?
One cup of orange juice provides about 100 milligrams of vitamin C—more than the RDA. There are also many other fruits and vegetables rich in this antioxidant. It is therefore quite easy to get more than the RDA of vitamin C through diet alone.

Vitamin E
What does vitamin E do?
- It helps prevent damage to cell membranes.
- It can detoxify free radicals (destructive substances that are by-products sometimes formed by body cells when oxygen is metabolized or burned).
- It helps heal body tissue and aids in the growth of new tissue.

How much do women over 50 need?
The current RDA for vitamin E is 8 milligrams for adult women of all ages; 150 percent of that would be 12 milligrams and 200 percent of the RDA would be 16 milligrams. (To convert from the older method of measuring vitamin E [IU] to the newer method [mg], 10 milligrams equal about 15 IU.) The Alliance for Aging Research advises Americans to take 100 IU (67 mg). The 1968 RDA board initially recommended 20 milligrams daily for this unique antioxidant, but they ended up reducing that by more than half, partly because it is rather difficult to get this amount of vitamin E every day through food sources alone.

Why might older women need more than the RDA?
You might need more vitamin E in your later years for the following reasons:

- There is an age-related decline in the vitamin E content of several body tissues.
- If the need for antioxidants increases (to help reduce the risk of several chronic diseases), then the need for vitamin E would likewise increase.
- There may be a relationship between a vitamin E–rich diet (or taking vitamin E supplements) and a reduced risk of **atherogenesis** (the creation of plaque in the arteries), cancer, cataracts, and heart disease.
- Higher levels of vitamin E in the blood have been correlated with a reduced incidence of infectious diseases.
- With daily doses of vitamin E as high as 500 IU, cellular immunity in healthy elderly people appears to rival that of younger folks, but more investigation into this area is needed.

Further, our biological need for vitamin E also rises as our polyunsaturated fat intake rises (you need more of the antioxidant vitamin E to protect all those unsaturated fats from oxidation). Luckily, vitamin E is found in many of the monounsaturated-fat and polyunsaturated-fat vegetable oils, such as safflower and canola oil. But if you are eating a low-fat diet that includes twice the RDA for vitamin E (which would be 16 mg), there will be much more vitamin E left over to perform its other important antioxidant duties, since you won't need as much to protect all the extra unsaturated fats from oxidation.

There is also some evidence that environmental conditions such as air pollution may increase your need for vitamin E. Air pollutants such as nitrogen dioxide or ozone can initiate damaging free-radical reactions, and vitamin E helps prevent these from occurring. (For more information on vitamin E, see chapter 8.)

Where do we get it?
You will take in just over 12 IU of vitamin E if you do all these things each day: eat two slices of whole-wheat bread, consume a total of 1 tablespoon of canola oil, drink 1 cup of orange juice, eat 1 cup of oatmeal, eat 1 cup of fresh, chopped spinach, eat one carrot, and eat 1 cup of cooked broccoli. Needless to say, even on a good day, this vitamin is a little hard to get a lot of—unless you're in the habit of using lots of vegetable oil or eating lots of high-fat seeds and nuts (which contain vitamin E). Thus, it is very difficult to get more than the RDA without taking a supplement.

(Note: High doses of vitamin E may interfere with anticlotting drugs. So if you're taking this type of medicine, consult your doctor before starting to take vitamin E supplements. And some studies show that extremely high amounts of vitamin E, 500 milligrams [800 IU] taken every day, can also cause nausea, weakness, headache, diarrhea, and fatigue in some people.)

Beta-Carotene
What does beta-carotene do?
The body can convert beta-carotene, along with other carotenoids, to vitamin A, which has many important functions:

- It is vital to eye function and prevents night blindness.
- It is essential for healthy skin and helps maintain cell membranes, such as the linings of the mouth, lungs, stomach, and the intestinal and urinary tracts.
- It plays a role in the body's immune system and in the growth of bones.
- It helps manufacture red blood cells and maintain the sheaths that surround nerve cell fibers.

How much do women over 50 need?
The current RDA for vitamin A, which includes beta-carotene, is 800 retinal equivalents (RE) for adult women. However, the Alliance for Aging Research advises Americans to take amounts much larger than that: about 5,100 RE, or retinal equivalents.

Why might older women need more than the RDA?
There is some evidence that antioxidants such as beta-carotene help slow the aging process, in part by helping protect the body against such chronic diseases as heart disease and cancer.

Where do we get it?
You will consume more than twice the recommended daily amount just by chewing on one average-sized carrot, which has roughly 2,000 RE. Other good sources of beta-carotene are sweet potatoes ($\frac{1}{2}$ cup of mashed sweet potatoes contains 1,900 RE); fresh spinach (1 cup contains 450 RE); and broccoli (1 cup has 220 RE). That morning tradition of a cup of orange juice will add 50 RE to your daily total. Thus, it is not difficult to get more than the RDA of beta-carotene from food sources.

Vitamin B-6
What does vitamin B-6 do?
- It plays an important role in protein and energy metabolism (in fact, your need for it increases as your intake of protein increases).
- It helps produce red blood cells and build certain amino acids. (It's also needed to convert some of these amino acids to hormones.)
- It is important in the function of nerve tissue.

How much do women over 50 need?
The current RDA for vitamin B-6 is 1.6 milligrams for adult women; 150 percent of that would be 2.4 milligrams. In a series of recent experiments, 1.9 to 2.3 milligrams was the amount needed to improve some areas of immune function.

Why might older women need more than the RDA?
A recent clinical study found that intakes higher than the RDA were necessary to keep vitamin B-6 at normal levels in elderly people. According to one researcher, 120 to 145 percent of the current RDA (which would be 1.9 to 2.3 mg) was needed to maintain a strong immune system.

Where do we get it?
Even the best sources of vitamin B-6 don't have a lot of it. A serving of instant oatmeal that has been fortified with vitamin B-6 has only 0.7 milligram. Two slices of whole-wheat bread contribute only 0.1 milligram. A cup of cooked beans contains from 0.2 to 0.3 milligram. And a roasted chicken breast provides only 0.5 milligram. Since it's difficult to get more than the RDA of this vitamin from food, supplements are necessary. But if you take a multivitamin-mineral supplement, it will usually contribute 100 percent of the RDA.

Vitamin B-12
What does vitamin B-12 do?
- It helps manufacture red blood cells.
- It helps maintain the sheaths around nerve cell fibers.

How much do women over 50 need?
The current RDA for vitamin B-12 is 2 micrograms (µg) for adult women.

Why might older women need more than the RDA?
Some studies have noted that while older people's consumption of this nutrient was generous, their blood levels were below normal. Many researchers listed B-12 as a vitamin whose RDA might increase after age 50. Those with less gastric acid being secreted from the stomach (about 30 percent of people over age 60) should definitely consume more than the RDA, because people with this disorder aren't absorbing as much vitamin B-12 into the bloodstream from the intestines.

Where do we get it?
Vitamin B-12 comes from animal products. One cup of skim milk provides almost half the recommended amount, with 0.9 microgram. Two ounces of reduced-fat cheese contain 0.5 microgram, 3 ounces of chicken breast pro-

vide 0.3 microgram, and a 3-ounce ground-sirloin burger will give you a whopping 1.7 microgram. It's only difficult to get more than the RDA of this vitamin from food if you're a strict vegetarian.

Vitamin D
What does vitamin D do?
- It influences the growth of strong bones by regulating calcium and phosphorus metabolism.
- It increases the amount of calcium actually absorbed by the body.
- It helps regulate some immune system functions.

How much do women over 50 need?
The current RDA for vitamin D is 200 IU (or 5 μg) for adult women. However, some researchers have suggested intakes of 400 IU for older people.

Why might older women need more than the RDA?
Aging decreases the capacity of the skin and kidneys to produce usable forms of vitamin D. Moreover, some studies have found that the aging intestine is less responsive to vitamin D. More vitamin D may be needed to help compensate for this deficiency. Another study showed that when 400 IU of vitamin D (twice the RDA) were given to healthy postmenopausal women, they had a net increase in the weight of the spinal bone over the 1-year experimental period.

Where do we get it?
Vitamin D is very rare in food (there is a little in some fish and eggs), so the foods that contain the most vitamin D are the ones that are fortified with it, like milk and some cereals. One cup of any fortified milk contains 100 IU, and a teaspoon of margarine contains 15 IU, and an ounce of cold cereal often contain 50 IU. One cooked egg contains 23 IU. Thus, you can get more than the RDA of this vitamin from food if you drink enough skim milk every day.

(Note: Taking too much vitamin D in *supplement* form—three to five times the RDA or more—can be toxic to the system.)

Folic Acid (Folate)
What does folic acid do?
- It is essential for DNA and RNA formation, which makes it especially important for bone marrow and the intestinal tract, where cell turnover is highest.
- It is required for the synthesis and breakdown of amino acids (protein building blocks).

How much do women over 50 need?

The current RDA is 180 micrograms for adult women. The more researchers know about folic acid, the more it appears it is a vitamin that helps protect the body from cellular damage and some disease. In the future, the RDA for this vitamin may be increased for the entire population.

Why might older women need more than the RDA?

A recent study reported in the *Journal of the Canadian Dietetic Association* found that, although older people's consumption of folic acid was generous, their blood levels were below normal. This means that your body's ability to absorb folic acid may decrease as you age. Lower amounts of folic acid in body tissues have also been associated with a higher risk of **cervical dysplasia** (abnormal cervical cell growth that is considered precancerous). There is also increasing evidence that folic acid acts much like an antioxidant by influencing the immune system and your body's ability to ward off cancer. And for a substantial number of older people with **gastric atrophy** (a shrinking and wasting of the stomach), some of the folate from food is not getting absorbed via the intestinal tract. For all these reasons, women in their later years should try to get more than the current recommended daily amount of folic acid.

In addition, according to Harvard Medical School researchers, folic acid may be one of the key ingredients in fruits and vegetables that helps prevent colon cancer by possibly assisting in the process that turns cancer genes off. Although claims that folic acid enhances many aspects of immunity are still not universally accepted, getting at least the recommended daily amount of folic acid from fruits and vegetables is without question a good way to help keep our immune system strong.

Where do we get it?

Folic acid is found in leafy green vegetables and beans. For example, 1 cup of broccoli has 78 micrograms, 1 cup of fresh spinach has 109 micrograms. A cup of cooked beans will give you anywhere from 120 to 300 micrograms. Oranges are also rich in folic acid: 1 cup of orange juice provides 109 micrograms. So it's not difficult to get more than the RDA of this vitamin from food if you eat all your vegetables.

Calcium

What does calcium do?

- It makes the bones and teeth strong. Ninety-nine percent of all the body's calcium is in the bones and teeth.
- It is necessary for nerve transmission, blood clotting, and to help regulate contractions such as the rythmic beating of the heart muscle.

- It is important in the function of several enzymes and in the absorption of vitamin B-12.

How much do women over 50 need?

The current RDA for calcium is 800 milligrams for women 25 years and older (1,200 mg for women age 19 to 24.) But recently the National Institutes of Health appointed a Consensus Development Panel on Optimal Calcium Intake, and that panel recommended 1,500 milligrams a day for postmenopausal women between age 50 and 64 not on estrogen or hormone replacement therapy, and for all women over 65. The panel also recommended 1,000 milligrams for postmenopausal women between 50 and 64 currently on hormone replacdment therapy.

Why might older women need more than the RDA?

After menopause, bone density decreases even faster than it did before menopause. Since calcium strengthens bones, this would be reason enough to increase your daily intake of it. In addition, however, calcium is not fully absorbed from the intestinal tract in our later years, so you habe to take in more of it for your body to be able to use as much as it did in the past.

Where do we get it?

If you don't mind several servings a day of dairy foods, getting 1,000 milligrams of calcium through your diet shouldn't be much trouble. But getting the amount recommended for women over 50 not on hormone replacement therapy, 1,500 milligrams, might require that you take a supplement. A cup of skim milk contains 302 milligrams, 2 ounces of reduced fat cheese contain 414 milligrams, a cup of lowfat fruit yogurt contains 345 milligrams, and a cup of broccoli adds 72 milligrams to the daily total. Getting more than the RDA from food, therefore, requires consuming a fair amount of low- or nonfat dairy products.

Chromium

What does chromium do?

- It is involved in carbohydrate and fat metabolism.
- It helps maintain blood sugar levels and possibly participates in insulin's action in the body.

How much do women over 50 need?

Currently there is no RDA for chromium. However, the RDA committee believes a safe and adequate daily intake is 50 to 200 micrograms.

Why might older women need more than this?

Body stores of chromium decline across our life span. This might be explained by declining amounts of chromium in our diet or our bodies may not metabolize chromium as well when we age. But chromium is still important in our later years. Among other things, it is essential for glucose (the simplest form of carbohydrate) metabolism. In fact, it has been suggested that adult-onset diabetes may be related in some way to a chromium deficiency.

Where do we get it?
The general rule about chromium is that the more refined or processed foods you eat, the less chromium you'll be getting. The most common food sources of chromium, besides whole grains and unrefined foods, are seafood, meat, nuts, cheeses, fats, vegetable oils, and some vegetables. Unfortunately, little information is available on the amount of chromium per serving of specific foods. But an estimated 90 percent of U.S. adults take in less than the suggested minimum of 50 micrograms. All of the vitamin-mineral supplements included in the table later in this chapter contain chromium (see Table 5.2).

Zinc
What does zinc do?
- It is required for the metabolism of protein, carbohydrates, fats and alcohol.
- It is necessary for the synthesis of DNA and RNA.
- It is required by over 70 enzymes as a **cofactor** (a mineral that works with an enzyme to facilitate chemical reactions).
- It is needed for immune response, healing wounds, and tissue growth and repair.
- It is needed to produce the active form of vitamin A.
- It participates in the production and removal of carbon dioxide at the cellular level.
- It is essential for tasting the saltiness in food.

How much do women over 50 need?
The current RDA for zinc is 12 milligrams for adult women.

Why might older women need more than the RDA?
First, zinc is not fully absorbed from the intestinal tract in our later years. One study, reported in the *Journal of the Canadian Dietetic Association,* noted that while older people's consumption of this nutrient was generous, their blood levels were below normal. Second, the immune system weakens as we grow older, and zinc is essential for a strong immune system. In fact, some researchers suspect that immune deficiency in older people may be due in part to the zinc deficiency commonly observed in older adults. Studies have proven that correcting a zinc deficiency can improve immune response and loss of taste, both symptoms of zinc deficiency. The improvements seemed to take place with 30 milligrams, which is over two times the RDA.

However, consuming over 100 milligrams may be harmful. This level of zinc can actually suppress your immune function, cause a copper deficiency and anemia, and lower your HDL ("good" cholesterol) level.

Where do we get it?
Zinc is a little more hard to get than some of the other minerals. Even the better food sources of zinc don't contain very much. The best sources are lean meat (a 3-ounce chicken breast contains 1 mg, 3 ounces of lean sirloin provide 4 mg); seafood (clams, crabs and oysters contain the most, but more everyday fish choices like sole or cod contain 0.5 mg per 3-ounce portion, while half a can of water-packed tuna contains 0.6 mg); whole grains, (two slices of whole-wheat bread and a cup of oatmeal each contain 1 mg); and beans (a cup of beans provides about 2 mg).

HOW TO GET THE VITAMINS AND MINERALS YOU NEED

The simple answer many of us hope for is to take an assortment of pills packed with these sought-after nutrients. Unfortunately, pills are *not* the best way to ensure that you're getting all the vitamins and minerals you need. What are the best ways?

1. Eat a balanced diet.
2. Take one complete, balanced vitamin-mineral supplement daily.

A variety of sensible foods from the major food groups should provide all the nutrients essential for good health. In particular, if you make four simple, specific food choices each and every day, you'll be closer to your goal of a balanced diet—just from these four simple food choices. Table 5.1 shows these four food choices and which of the ten key vitamins and minerals they contain. The only nutrients from the 10 most-wanted list that *aren't* provided by these four food choices are zinc and vitamin B-6 (and vitamin E in large amounts).

Table 5.1. Four Foods to Better Nutrition

Food Choice	Vitamins and Minerals You'll Get
1 cup of broccoli or 1 cup of fresh chopped spinach	Vitamin C, vitamin E, beta-carotene, folic acid, and calcium
1 carrot	Beta-carotene and a little vitamin E and folic acid
1 cup of orange juice	Vitamin C, beta-carotene, and folic acid
1 cup of skim milk	Vitamin B-12, vitamin D, and calcium

WHAT ABOUT VITAMIN-MINERAL SUPPLEMENTS?

While you can get most of the vitamins and minerals you need through food sources, the reality is that most Americans don't come close to meeting the basic dietary recommendations. Many of us, therefore, want to take a vitamin-mineral supplement to make up the balance. In fact, nearly half of the women in the United States routinely use some vitamin-mineral supplement. (Indeed, whenever I hear health care professionals weighing the pros and cons of taking vitamin-mineral supplements, I always ask, "But do you take one?" Usually the answer is yes.)

Vitamin-mineral supplements are tempting; they epitomize America's propensity for quick fixes: We love the idea of popping a pill to cure our ills. We also like to think that if a little is good, a lot must be better. The problem is, nutritionally speaking, both these ideas are usually untrue.

Almost all health professionals agree that dietary supplements are no substitute for a healthy diet and lifestyle. A vitamin-mineral supplement isn't going to make a high-fat diet any lower in fat or a low-fiber diet any higher in fiber. Nonetheless, vitamin-mineral supplements should be considered for special groups who may have a difficult time meeting their bodies' nutrient requirements through food sources alone. These groups include growing children, people on weight-reduction diets, and pregnant women. Women in or after menopause might also benefit from a balanced and complete vitamin-mineral supplement, given that many women in this group start eating less (in response to their decreased metabolism) at the same time that their needs for some nutrients start increasing.

So, if you are looking for a vitamin-mineral supplement to help you through menopause and beyond, you should know which supplements are best for you and have safe and sensible doses. See Table 5.2 for a description of the seven best supplements.

Getting the Most from Vitamin-Mineral Supplements

There are shopping carts full of vitamin-mineral supplements on the market. Here are some guidelines to help you evaluate and get the most benefit from a vitamin-mineral supplement.

Be sure it's complete.
Select a vitamin-mineral supplement that has a complete array of vitamins and minerals. Nutrients work together, so it's best to choose a supplement that includes a mix of all the essential ones. A complete supplement should contain all these vitamins and minerals with established RDAs: all the B vitamins (thiamin, riboflavin, niacin, vitamin B-6, folic acid, vitamin B-12,

Table 5.2. The Seven Best Vitamin-Mineral Supplements for Menopause and Beyond

Brand	Average Cost per Month	Complete	Balanced	Calcium (% RDA)	Iron (% RDA)	Beta-Carotene
ABC to Z (Nature's Bounty)	$1.50	Yes	Yes	16%	100%	Yes*
Centrum	$3.50	Yes	Yes	16%	100%	20% of vitamin A total
Myadec	$2.80	Yes	Yes	16%	100%	25%
One-A-Day Maximum	$3.85	Yes	Yes	13%	100%	0–50%
Sentral-Vite (K-mart)	$1.15	Yes	Yes	16%	100%	25%
Spectrovite (Pathmark)	$1.20	Yes	Yes	16%	100%	Yes
Vita-Lea (Shaklee)	$11.15	Yes**	Yes	60%	100%	No

This table reflects data as of September 1994.

*Exact amount not available from manufacturer.

**This supplement met all the rules except one: It doesn't contain any beta-carotene. I included it anyway because it contains the most calcium of all the supplements that made the table.

biotin, pantothenic acid); vitamins A, C, D, and E; and the minerals calcium, copper, iodine, iron, magnesium, phosphorus, and zinc. Although there isn't an RDA established for the mineral chromium, you might also make sure your supplement contains the minimum amount suggested by the RDA committee, at least 50 micrograms, since it's one of the minerals that we might need more of as we age.

Be sure it's balanced.
Look for a balanced nutrient profile, with the supplement providing close to 100 percent of the RDA for most of the vitamins and minerals. However, you'll find that biotin isn't usually present at this level, because it is particularly expensive. Nor are calcium and magnesium normally present at this

level either, because they are so bulky that the pills would be too large to swallow.

Many nutrients can cause medical problems—or, at the very least, discomfort—at excessive doses. See Table 5.3 for specific risks you should be aware of. High doses of some vitamins or minerals can also knock out the benefits of others. For example, high doses of zinc interfere with your body's absorption of copper. So unless you have a specific reason for doing so and know it's safe, avoid consuming more than 100 percent of vitamins and minerals (except perhaps vitamin E) in supplement form.

Look for some calcium but not too much iron.

American women have a tendency to eat less than the recommended amounts of these two minerals, so your supplement must contain both calcium and iron, but not too much iron. The amount of calcium in the supplements listed in Table 5.2 ranges from 13 to 60 percent of the RDA (though most provide 16 percent). All the supplements listed provide exactly 100 percent of the RDA for iron. Supplements that contain much larger amounts of iron were left out of the table because too much iron can cause health problems, especially for postmenopausal women and 10 percent of the population that are genetically prone to "iron overload." Because your body can't rid itself of excess iron, it accumulates in tissues and organs. This stockpiling can result in irreversible arthritis, diabetes, and heart irregularities. Men and postmenopausal women, whose iron requirements are lower, are the most susceptible to iron overload.

Look for some beta-carotene.

In most cases, if there is any beta-carotene in a vitamin-mineral supplement, it is included in the vitamin A total, since the body is able to form vitamin A from beta-carotene. Most of the vitamin companies are not yet listing on their labels what portion of the vitamin A percent RDA is coming from beta-carotene. (If the label is unclear, you can call the company directly.) Ideally, more of the vitamin A total should come from beta-carotene. Vitamin A is a fat-soluble vitamin and, at higher levels, can accumulate in the body and become potentially toxic. On the other hand, beta-carotene is a water-soluble substance, and the body is able to get rid of any excess.

Look for a supplement that takes no longer than 30 minutes to disintegrate.

In order for your body to be able to absorb and use the vitamins and minerals contained in your supplement, the pill must first dissolve while it is in your stomach or small intestine. If it takes longer than about 30 minutes to dissolve, the tablet will pass through you and end up supplementing the sewer

Table 5.3. Potential Risks from Excessive Supplementary Doses of Selected Minerals and Vitamins

Nutrient	Excessive Levels of Supplemental Daily Dose	Potential Risks
Minerals		
Calcium	> 3,000 mg	Constipation, confusion, urinary stone formation (in susceptible people), interference with iron absorption
Iron	N/A (specific amounts are not available)	Accidental poisoning (in children), constipation, clogging of the arteries
Niacin	> 10× the RDA	Liver damage, abnormal gastrointestinal function, painful tingling caused by dilated capillaries, peptic ulcers, laboratory evidence of diabetes
Selenium	> 1 mg (the RDA is 0.055 mg)	Vomiting or diarrhea, loss of hair and nails, lesions of skin and nervous system, altered cholesterol metabolism and blood lipid levels, accelerating atherosclerosis
Zinc	> 3–10× the RDA	Impaired immune response, reduced copper absorption, anemia, lowered levels of HDL ("good") cholesterol
Vitamins		
Vitamin A	> 10× the RDA (prolonged use)	Birth defects, severe liver damage, headaches, vomiting, bone damage, diarrhea
Vitamin B-6	> 1 g (prolonged use) 625× the RDA	Serious nerve disorders, including numbness and muscle weakness
Vitamin C	> 2 g (but especially at levels of 8 g a day)	Diarrhea, urinary-tract abnormalities
Vitamin D	> 3× the RDA	Irreversible kidney, heart, and blood vessel damage; bone malformation
Folic acid	> 1 mg	Masks symptoms of vitamin B-12 deficiency

instead. All the supplements I've included in Table 5.2 meet the disintegration standards proposed by U.S. Pharmacopeia (USP), the scientific organization that establishes drug standards. Such supplements disintegrate completely within 30 to 45 minutes.

Don't buy a supplement that is past its expiration date.
Just as different foods can go bad, some faster than others, so can vitamins. The vitamins more sensitive to heat, air, and time, can lose their potency. In order to maximize the effectiveness of your vitamins, therefore, take them before the expiration date stamped on the bottle.

Be wary of botanicals in supplements.
Some supplements include various botanical substances. Remember, though, that if you take a botanical supplement, you do so at your own risk. Don't use herbal remedies for serious illnesses like heart disease, cancer or arthritis without consulting your doctor or nurse practitioner. There are known risks involved with taking too much of some herbal supplements. For instance:

- **Chapparal** can cause toxic hepatitis.
- **Comfrey** can cause liver disease.
- **Germanium** can cause irreversible kidney damage, even death.
- **Gums** can cause intestinal blockages, diarrhea, and bloating.
- **Jin bu huan** can depress the central nervous system in children and has caused deaths.
- **Ma huang** can cause high blood pressure, nerve damage, and muscle injury, and is particularly unsafe if you have heart disease, diabetes, or thyroid disease.
- **Yohimbe** can cause tremors, anxiety, high blood pressure, rapid heart rate, kidney failure, seizures, and death.

Don't take supplements on an empty stomach.
Take your supplement with or after a meal, when it has a better chance of being dissolved and absorbed. This is because many of the vitamins and minerals are more likely to be absorbed in the presence of other nutrients—for example, iron in the presence of vitamin C, or calcium in the presence of vitamin D and magnesium.

Talk with your health care provider.
Tell your doctor or nurse practitioner about all the supplements you take, to avoid unwanted interactions with other medications. Certain medications might render your supplements useless or certain supplements could make your medication less effective.

FOOD FIRST

Although some vitamin-mineral supplements may be necessary for menopausal and postmenopausal women, food must still come first on your list of priorities. Nature made it complete and balanced. Supplementation, on the other hand, hasn't yet been studied extensively enough. There are still many important questions unanswered. The truth is that we have not yet discovered enough about all the phytochemicals and other beneficial substances in foods, to be able to reproduce them in pill form. Nor do we know all there is to know about how nutrients work in combination with one another to enhance health and prevent disease. So your safest bet (and, incidentally, also the most economical) is still food, especially unprocessed or minimally processed. If you eat a balanced, healthy diet, you don't have to wait for scientists to discover every single phytochemical or important nutrient combination—you're already getting them!

LOOKING YOUNG: WEIGHT-LOSS WISDOM FOR MENOPAUSE AND BEYOND

Given the facts most menopausal women are facing about their declining metabolic rate and expanding waistline, your impulse may be to turn to quick weight-loss diets or programs. *Don't do it!* They don't work. But that doesn't mean you have to resign yourself to unwanted bulges and a rapidly expanding waistline. There are practical steps you can take to discourage unwanted weight gain. And the great part of it is, these steps are beneficial toward your health in general—preventing chronic diseases, generating more energy, and helping you feel better about yourself.

Do You Really Need to Lose Weight?

Ask yourself what you are really trying to achieve and why. What's driving your desire to lose or maintain your weight—peer or spousal pressure, media images, the mirror, changes in how your clothes fit, or health concerns? And isn't it extra body fat that you're trying to lose rather than just generic pounds?

Consider this: Muscle weighs more than fat, so don't give your scale any power. In fact, you may want to put your scale away in a closet. That may sound drastic, but you're better off without it. How you feel and what you look like without your clothes on are far better indicators of the appropriateness of your weight. (And besides, a weight scale is only a doctor's visit away.) Then, if you exercise regularly and take steps to eat healthily, you'll start feeling better about how you look. You'll start building more lean body mass and burning more excess body fat. Your clothes may even begin to fit better.

Don't Catch the Dieting Fever

Fad dieting is like gambling. When people catch the dieting fever, it doesn't matter what their past experience has taught them—all good sense goes out the window. All they can focus on is how this particular quick weight-loss product or program is different. This is the salvation from cellulite they'd been hoping for!

Let's start with some cold, hard facts. The success rates of the *best* weight-loss treatments available are disturbingly low. Even the promoters of many of the very low-calorie diets admit that only a minority of their patients end up maintaining the weight loss over the long term. A large study, reported in the *International Journal of Obesity*, followed over 4,000 patients who had used the Optifast program, a popular liquid diet providing 420 calories per day. After 18 months, only 12 percent of those who seriously committed themselves to the program had maintained their weight loss.

Here are some other cold, hard facts.

1. *Very low-calorie diets cost you some muscle.*   Obese subjects, after following a very low-calorie diet, often lose 3 to 6 percent of their body's muscle. But after they gain the weight back, all the muscle previously lost is *not* replaced. Some experts believe that this net muscle loss may contribute to lower calorie requirements and thus subsequent easy weight gain. So if you want to conserve as much of your muscle as possible, avoid very low-calorie diets (less than 800 calories per day) or other similar diets where you lose more than 3 or 4 pounds per week.

2. *You'll likely be down, up, down, and up again.*   Roller coasters are great fun at amusement parks but new research shows that riding the weight-loss roller coaster—where you lose 30 to 50 pounds, then gain them back (or more), down again, and up again—can seriously distort the body's weight regulation system, creating quite an ironic predicament: The more diets you go on, the harder it becomes to lose weight. (Sound familiar?) You may actually get to a point where you lose little weight even when on a near-starvation diet. So unless you are prepared to *permanently* change your bad eating habits and sedentary lifestyle, it may do more harm than good to lose pounds only to regain them. Not only does weight cycling seem to make future weight loss physiologically more difficult and future weight gain more easy, but some experts believe that these extreme fluctuations in body weight may themselves increase the risk for coronary heart disease—in addition to the risk due to obesity.

3. *There are major downfalls to diet pills.*   Phenylpropanolamine (PPA), an alleged appetite suppressant, is one of the more common diet aide ingredients. In a recently published study, the average weight loss of people taking PPA over a 6-week period was only 2 pounds greater than those receiving a placebo (something that looks like medicine but is really an inactive substance like sugar). That's not too terribly impressive for something

that costs an arm and a leg, should only be taken for up to 12 weeks, and can cause such side effects as dizziness, headaches, rapid pulse, palpitations, sleeplessness, and hypertension. *Don't take diet pills.* The minimal benefits they may offer in no way justify their considerable risks.

So What's a Weight/Body-Conscious Woman to Do?

Here's the answer: Shed the most fat while sacrificing the least amount of muscle. There are three parts to this solution:

1. Lower your daily intake of calories by just 200 to 300.
2. Eat a low-fat (not a no-fat) diet.
3. Gradually increase the frequency and duration of your exercise.

Of course, there's a little more to it than that, but basically that's the ticket. And guess what? Many of the practical steps you can take to encourage body fat loss are already part of the 10 Diet Commandments. So by following the good-sense diet advice in this book, you should find yourself feeling healthier and better about your body as well.

The Western Human Nutrition Research Center-USDA Agricultural Research Service, which is located in San Francisco, studied the effects that two types of dieting measures had on moderately overweight women. One group followed a moderate-calorie diet (cutting 25 percent of their calories) and a moderate exercise program (which increased their calorie needs by 25 percent). The other group endured a more drastic low-calorie diet (cutting 50 percent of their calories) but *without* any exercise. And guess what the lower-calorie dieters got for their trouble? They lost the same amount of actual body fat as the moderate-calorie dieters who also exercised.

In a recent Purdue University study, dieters participating in a weight-loss program who had supportive partners (not in the program) dropped up to 30 percent more weight during a 15-month period than those who flew solo. And "supportive" seems to be the operative factor here (not just having a partner), because if the dieter's partner gained weight during the period, the dieter was likely to gain as well.

Though your need for many vitamins and minerals increases during and after menopause, your calories needs shrink (due to hormonal changes affecting your metabolism). So, more than ever, you need to eat foods that provide the maximum amounts of vitamins and minerals with the fewest calories. And, more than ever, you need to exercise and eat right to raise your metabolic rate. Finally, our bodies, no matter what our age, like to use carbohydrates for everyday energy and prefer to store extra fat calories—as fat. So, to keep your body happy, eat lots of carbohydrates—and less fat.

Have a Healthy Relationship with Food

Some think dieting puts them in control of their weight and eating habits. In reality, though, it's the other way around: Dieting and food control them. Indeed, it's the very rigidity of restrained eating that leads many people to eventually lose control. So your first task is to commit yourself to no more dieting and no more forbidden foods. We know now that deprivation feeds bingeing, and bingeing feeds guilt, and guilt feeds the dieting impulse, which then leads to more deprivation and more bingeing. And the frustrating, self-defeating cycle goes on and on.

Let's get back to the basics. Food is a good thing; food is nourishment. Eating is supposed to be an enjoyable experience, often shared with friends and family. Don't let your fear of food or fear of fat blind you from these basic truths. Healthy food can be enjoyed, too—especially if it is eaten in a general spirit of health and happiness.

6

EATING FOR ENERGY

Being healthy doesn't just mean being free from illness. It means sleeping well and being alert when awake, full of life and energy, able to move around easily—and *wanting* to move around, for that matter. It's the difference between feeling good and feeling great. When the proverbial "How are you?" is asked, good health is the difference between automatically responding, "Fine," and exclaiming, "Terrific!" That's what this chapter is all about: achieving that higher level of health and energy so that you can feel fabulous and perform at your peak at whatever you choose to do.

FOOD: YOUR ENERGY SOURCE

Food is your body's fuel source. So one of the best ways to boost your energy level is to give your body the best possible fuel—the healthiest food. Give your body what it needs, when it need it; prime it with exercise to use that fuel well—and you'll be on your way to higher-energy living.

Making Calories Work *for*, Not Against You

When many women even hear the word "calorie," red flags start flapping, and buzzers start going off, because may women fear that "calorie" means "weight gain." Not true. A calorie is first and foremost a measurement of how much energy a substance has.

Just as cars need gasoline to run their engines, people need calories to run their bodies. There are only four sources of calories in our diet: carbohydrates, protein, fat and alcohol. Of These, our bodies are designed to use carbohydrate calories for most of our energy needs. Protein is used mainly as a builder of muscle, enzymes, or hormones. Fat is used for storing calories; it is also a source of fat-soluble vitamins and essential fatty acids. Alcohol is essentially good for nothing: Your body considers it a toxic substance and tries to get rid of it (via the kidneys and lungs) or metabolize it as quickly as possible. When consumed in excess of your energy needs, alcohol calories are converted to body fat.

To keep your body fueled with energy, not only do you need the right *number* of calories, but you also need the right *type* of calories—that is, mostly carbohydrates. And you need these calories to hit your bloodstream at the right *times*.

Getting the Right Amount of Calories

Some experts calculate that a moderately active woman needs at least 1,800 calories a day to meet her energy needs and maintain her weight. But how much does a moderately active woman need if she's in the midst of menopause need? Your metabolism starts slowing down as you age and following menopause. Many women find it more and more difficult to lose unwanted extra pounds during and after menopause (and, unfortunately, easier and easier to collect unwanted pounds.) Most menopausal women gain an average of 12 pounds, and even more important, their body fat increases an average of 1 to 4 percent.

While genetics do affect how your body will handle extra calories, menopause is one of the cases where almost everyone, thin or plump, needs to be aware of ways to prevent weight gain. A recent study, published in *Archives of Internal Medicine*, showed that both thin women and overweight women gained about the same number of pounds between the ages of 42 and 53. In fact, the researchers found that most women experienced considerable weight gain during their forties. They suggest that this is due to the age-related reduction in metabolic rate or the drop in physical activity that tends to accompany older age. The amount of physical activity is, of course, a factor you can control to some extent. Significantly, the women in the study who had the lowest exercise levels gained the most weight.

I won't explain here how you can calculate your optimal calorie needs, because the individual determinates vary too widely from woman to woman. And I don't even want to encourage you to count calories every day because it fuels the fire of self-restriction and diet obsession, something this country has too much of already. Instead, you can figure that if you are currently maintaining your weight, you are probably getting approximately the right number of calories. If you are currently gaining extra weight in the form of fat, then perhaps you should decrease your caloric intake slightly. (You can estimate your current caloric intake using the exercises in chapter 10.) But you might be better served by reducing your fat intake first, especially if your average intake of calories from fat proves to be more than 30 percent of your total calorie intake, and by increasing your activity level. (Exercise 8 in chapter 10 shows how to calculate the percentage of calories from fat in your diet.)

Getting the Right Type of Calories

The government's recommendations for the general population are to consume about 60 percent of one's daily calories from carbohydrates, 15 percent from protein, and less than 30 percent calories from fat. There are many reasons why the majority of our daily calories should come from carbohydrates. One reason is that several of the major organs prefer to use carbohydrates for energy; some other reasons have to do with the health hazards of taking in too much of the other two energy sources, protein and fat.

Carbohydrates: The Perfect Energy Food

Why are carbohydrates the fuel of choice? Because all body cells can readily utilize **glucose,** which is the major substance produced when carbohydrates are broken down in the body. In fact, the red blood cells and the central nervous system (which includes your brain), actually function better when carbohydrates are their fuel source. In addition, carbohydrates play an essential role in metabolizing fat: You need carbohydrates to use fat for energy.

What are these prefered carbohydrates, and where can you find them? Carbohydrates come in two basic food packages—sugars and starches, both of which are found in plants and in some dairy products. Sugars are the smallest and simplest of the carbohydrates, and typically taste sweet. Starches are called **complex carbohydrates** because they have much larger molecules made up of many sugar units linked together. You'll find these complex carbohydrates in plant seeds, roots, tubers, grains, nuts, legumes, root vegetables, and potatoes. Fruits are primarily composed of **simple carbohydrates** (or simple sugars).

The last piece to the carbohydrate puzzle is fiber. Fiber is actually made up of linked carbohydrate units. But, since it cannot be digested by the human gastrointestinal tract, it cannot be absorbed, and therefore cannot contribute calories. (For more information on fiber, see chapter 8.)

Why Not Eat More Protein?

The food protein you eat gets broken down into individual amino acids in your digestive tract. The body then uses these amino acids to make the proteins that are needed within the body. The body needs protein for growth and maintenance of its tissues, and synthesizing enzymes (proteins that stimulate chemical reactions in the body,) hormones (chemical messengers that travel to various target tissues or organs,) and antibodies. Proteins are also involved in blood clotting, fluid balance and acid-base balance within the body.

Yet if protein is so important, isn't eating more protein better? No. Remember that your cells use amino acids for energy only when they are forced to, when glucose or fatty acids are limited. Protein is the body's last choice as a fuel for energy. So if you eat protein in excess of your normal needs and your body doesn't need it for energy at that moment, your body will convert it to the ultimate form of energy storage, fat.

How Much Food Fat?

Fat has more than twice as many calories per gram (9) as either carbohydrates or protein (4 each). So why not just eat lots of fat for energy? This would work well if you were in danger of not getting enough food, but alas, most of us have plenty. Instead, you are more likely to be in need of more vitamins, minerals, and fiber than you are currently getting. And you're probably trying to reduce your body fat, especially if you're approaching and passing menopause. Unfortunately, nothing adds body fat faster than a high-fat diet.

When I did a computer analysis of typical high-fat and low-fat diets, I found that the benefits of a low-fat diet are that:

- It contains more vitamins and minerals and fiber.
- It gives you more energy.
- It helps diminish some menopausal symptoms.
- It helps prevent or reverse obesity.
- It helps prevent some cancers and heart disease.

After the traditional Thanksgiving feast, have you ever felt like the stuffed turkey? On the outside, you're unfastening your clothing, maybe making your way to the medicine cabinet in search of any way to spell relief. On the inside, your stomach has been stretched to its largest holding capacity. Well, when you eat a high-fat meal, a higher proportion of your blood supply is circulating to your stomach area (where food digestion takes place) for a longer period of time. And the more blood that's diverted into the stomach to help with digestion, the less blood is circulating to the rest of your body—carrying less oxygen to the brain and muscles. The brain gets a little slow without a full supply of oxygen, so you become sleepy.

The more fat in your meal, the longer food will hang around in your stomach. And the longer it's in the stomach, the longer some of your blood will be diverted to the stomach area (and not to your brain, and working muscles), and the longer you'll feel the food weighing you down. (Liquids, on the other hand, exit the stomach only 15 to 30 minutes after mealtime—that's why liquid diets don't satisfy you for long.) And fried foods are the worst. Fried foods are digested even more slowly than fatty foods prepared by other cooking methods, because the food particles coated with fat must be broken up into smaller pieces before the enzymes can work their digestive magic on them. That's why meals high in carbohydrate and low in fat are just plain easier on the stomach and leave you feeling more energetic after eating.

So what's the ideal target for fat consumption? The government's dietary guidelines tell us to eat less than 30 percent of our daily calories from fat. If you make sensible choices, it's easy enough to hit this target. You can still go to the same eating establishments (even fast-food restaurants), and you can still eat many of your favorite foods (even desserts). I've written three books helping people do just that. But what's best for menopausal and post-menopausal women? Some of the same cardiovascular benefits of an extremely low-fat diet (around 10 percent of total calories from fat) can be achieved with a diet that provides 20 percent of its calories from fat. Cancer prevention research seems to support that target, too. Obesity research also suggests an ideal of about 20 percent of total calories from fat for people who are trying to lose body fat or maintain their weight. For women over 40 or 50, a realistic goal would be to consume 20 to 25 percent of your total calories from fat. (See chapter 9 for information on how this translates into food terms.)

Indeed, if you are going to count anything, count fat. The University of Minnesota recently completed a study on women who weighed 20 to 40 percent over their ideal weight. Half the women followed weight-loss regimens in which they were told to eat no more than 1,200 calories a day and a maximum of 40 grams of fat (30 percent of total calories). The other group was told to eat as much of foods high in complex carbohydrates (fruits, vegetables, rice, pasta, beans, and bread) as it took to feel satisfied but were also instructed to gradually lower their fat intake to just 20 grams a day. What these two groups of women actually did was another matter altogether. The first group, the calorie counters, got down, on average, to 1,550 calories a day (the goal was 1,200). Meanwhile, the second group, the fat watchers, lowered their daily consumption of fat to an average of 37 grams (the goal was 20). But even while consuming 37 grams of fat, the fat counters lost the same amount of weight as the calorie counters: an average of 8 to 10 pounds during a 6-month period. But, more important, the fat counters scored higher on the quality-of-life measurements like general energy level and feelings of cheerfulness. And 6 months after the study was completed, the fat counters had kept 50 percent of their lost weight off, and still reported enjoying their food more. In contrast, the calorie counters had kept off only 20 percent of their lost weight.

Granted, there are lots of good reasons to eat a lowfat diet, including the likelihood of losing weight or maintaining your ideal weight. Nonetheless, there is still no guarantee that you will, in fact, lose weight. If you are eating low-fat foods or products, but eating too much of them or not exercising enough, it is possible your body will store some of those extra calories as body fat. *You still have to burn more energy through activity than you consume in calories* (from any source) if you want your body to use up its accumulated fat.

Getting Calories at the Right Times

Almost as important for energy and body fat balance as *what* you eat, is *when* you eat. Think about when your body needs energy the most; it makes sense for your meals to match your metabolic needs. Sure, many of us moms have told our children, "Breakfast is the most important meal of the day." But have we really thought about why? And do we practice what we preach?

Breakfast is actually *one* of the most important meals of the day. The other is lunch. Why are they so important? Because those are the times when we need to get the calories that are going to fuel us through the majority of our day. Depending on the exact composition and size of your meal, your blood glucose level peaks about $1\frac{1}{2}$ to 2 hours after eating; that is when you have the highest supply of immediate energy. We burn about 70 percent of all of our calories as fuel during the day time hours. But when do many American women eat the majority of their calories? During the *evening* hours. When you do this, you might be storing the majority of those calories as body fat because your body is metabolizing all those calories at a time when you are expending the *least* amount of energy (burning the fewest calories).

In one recent study, people were given one 2,000 calorie meal per day, either in the morning or in the evening. All the people in the breakfast group lost weight while four of the six people in the evening group gained weight.

So what you eat for breakfast is your fuel for what's ahead for the morning. What you eat for lunch is your fuel for the afternoon and early evening. And what you eat for dinner is really only fueling your night's sleep. Most of us start gearing down around dinnertime. We fold laundry, watch television, read stories to our children or grandchildren, return phone calls, and do other similarly gentle activities, none of which requires a whole lot of energy. And all of these evening activities are followed by sleep, when your basal metabolic rate (BMR) is at its lowest.

Why Eating Small and Frequent Meals Is Better

Eating more frequent meals is also an important way to match your metabolism. You need energy consistently throughout the day. By eating frequent, smaller meals, you are gently introducing the calories from carbohydrates, proteins, and fats into your bloodstream. This prevents wide swings in blood glucose so you don't feel tired when glucose levels drop. You also avoid quick elevations of blood lipids, a plus because high lipids increase the risk for heart disease.

Moreover, if you flood your bloodstream with too much fat, protein, and carbohydrates (meaning, in excess of your energy requirements at that moment), your body is going to have to dispose of those extra calories. Fats can be deposited in fat storage cells or in the arteries; carbohydrates can be converted to their storage form (glycogen) or converted to fat storage; and extra protein not used for muscle maintenance or synthesizing enzymes or hormones can eventually be converted to fat.

Small, frequent meals are also easier on the stomach and leave you more energetic after eating. Food will not stay as long in the stomach before proceeding to the intestines when you eat a high-carbohydrate, low-fat meal. So when you eat light, you can move around easier and you're not as sleepy. By eating small, frequent meals and snacks about every 3 to 4 hours, you will also be increasing your metabolism and maintaining your blood sugar level more easily, thereby avoiding that shaky, tired, irritable feeling that comes with blood sugar lows (**hypoglycemia**) for some people. This pattern also keeps us from getting overly hungry, which can lead to choosing the first foods you see (not necessarily the healthiest foods) or over-eating because once your blood sugar drops, nothing seems to satisfy your appetite.

These recommendations about the timing, frequency, and size of the meals you eat lead us to another Diet Commandment.

DIET COMMANDMENT #5

Eat Many Small Meals throughout the Day, and Eat Light at Night

---

Getting the Right Nutrients

Many vitamins and minerals also play a role in one very important energy component, your blood. Your body can't complete most energy-producing reactions without oxygen. Just as fire needs oxygen in order to burn, so the body needs oxygen in order to burn calories and produce energy. Oxygen binds with hydrogen and carbon from various energy sources to form carbon dioxide (CO_2), water (H_2O), and energy. And it is blood that carries oxygen, via the red blood cells, to where it's needed.

So keeping your red blood cells healthy and happy is essential for high-energy metabolism. (Metabolism can be defined as all the energy and material transformations that occur within living cells.) And several vitamins and minerals are necessary for the metabolic processes that produce energy. We'll look specifically at the minerals iron and zinc and vitamins A, C, and E. For these nutrients, among their other functions, either assist in metabolism directly or are components of enzymes essential for metabolism.

Iron

The greatest portion of iron in the body is in the hemoglobin of blood cells. Iron helps the hemoglobin carry oxygen to all cells in the body; it also helps transport carbon dioxide back to the lungs. It is also involved in energy metabolism. Indeed, one of the most common medical causes of fatigue is anemia, which refers to low blood levels of iron. Iron deficiency is easy to test for, so if it's a possibility, see your doctor. Sometimes even when blood hemoglobin tests *don't* indicate anemia, women may be suffering from low iron reserves. If you're not getting enough iron, the body depletes its iron reserves to maintain the blood's oxygen-carrying capacity.

Because iron is a component of blood, when women menstruate they lose some of their body's supply of iron. The Recommended Daily Allowance of iron decreases from 18 milligrams to 10 milligrams for women over 50 years of age, because generally these women have stopped menstruating. However, women over 50 should still be concerned about their iron intake. Since many women start eating fewer calories during this time of life, they need to make sure their diets include some of the best sources of iron. In fact, many recent studies have shown that it's the form more than the amount of dietary iron that influences our iron levels the most. And the form of iron that is most readily absorbed and therefore considered the best is lean red meat. Generally, a higher percentage of iron found in animal flesh foods (meat, fish, and poultry) is absorbed compared to the iron in eggs, milk, and plant foods.

However, we also know that eating too much meat isn't healthy. Luckily, there are two ways to increase the amount of iron that your body absorbs without eating more meat.

1. *Eat nonmeat sources of iron along with meat.* Eating iron sources in combination like this allows more of the nonmeat iron to be absorbed. Scientists observed that adding 3 ounces of meat, fish, or poultry to a meal can more than double the absorption of the nonmeat iron.
2. *Eat an iron-containing food with a vitamin C–rich food.* Vitamin C helps more of the iron be absorbed. Scientists found that adding 75 milligrams of vitamin C to a meal can at least double the amount of nonmeat iron absorbed from that meal. That's the amount of vitamin C in just 6 ounces of orange juice, $\frac{1}{2}$ cup of strawberries, or a cup of broccoli.

Best Food Choices for Iron: Lean meats, fish, poultry, legumes (dried beans and peas), nuts and seeds, whole grains and enriched grain products (pasta and rice), dark molasses, and leafy green vegetables.

Iron doesn't work by itself. A deficiency of vitamin B-6, vitamin E, folic acid, B-12, vitamins A or C, or copper can affect the hemoglobin level in the body and can indirectly create an iron deficiency. The following vitamins are also necessary for the production of red blood cells: vitamin B-2, riboflavin, vitamin B-6, vitamin B-12, and folic acid.

Zinc

Zinc, like iron, is important for high energy. Zinc is a constituent of the hormone insulin, which is responsible for the metabolism of excess blood sugar (glucose) and for maintaining proper blood sugar levels. It is also necessary for the metabolism of protein, carbohydrates, fat, and alcohol. Over 70 enzymes require zinc as a cofactor (a nonprotein substance that bind to an enzyme so that a desirable reaction can take place between the enzyme and another substance).

> *Best Food Choices for Zinc:*
> Seafood, lean meats, whole grains and legumes.

Vitamin A

Vitamin A boosts energy by assisting in the manufacture of red blood cells. It also helps ensure the normal production of thyroxin (a hormone that helps regulate metabolism) by the thyroid gland.

> *Best Food Choices for Vitamin A:* Dark green leafy and yellow/orange/red vegetables, some fruits (apricots, cantaloupe, mangoes, papaya), and margarines and milks that are fortified with vitamin A.

Vitamin C

Vitamin C increases energy by helping with the synthesis of thyroxin, which helps regulate metabolism.

> *Best Food Choices for Vitamin C:* Fruits (especially citrus fruits) and fresh vegetables (especially dark green vegetables).

Vitamin E

If the level of vitamin E in our blood falls too low, our red blood cells tend to break open, causing a form of anemia that results in fatigue. Some evidence suggests that environmental conditions like air pollution may increase our requirements for this vitamin.

> *Best Food Choices for Vitamin E:* Unrefined vegetable oils (like canola, soybean, sunflower, and corn), soybeans, tofu, lima beans, dark green leafy vegetables (dandelion greens, mustard and turnip greens, kale, and spinach), green vegetables (peas and asparagus), sweet potatoes, and whole grains (brown rice, whole-wheat bread, and oatmeal).

BOOSTING YOUR B VITAMINS—
THE ENERGY RELEASERS

If you take a quick perusal through the vitamin supplement aisle in your neighborhood supermarket or health food store, you'll notice that certain vitamin combinations are touted as special "energy-releasing" formulas. You'll usually find that the vitamins in those pills are mainly those referred to as "B complex" vitamins. While it's tempting to believe that these pills can give you more energy, their action is not quite that simple.

Carbohydrates, fats, and proteins are the substances used for energy or stored in the body as reserve fuel. But your body needs many vitamins, mainly B vitamins, in order to *convert* those substances to energy. In short, although you can't get energy from food without vitamins and minerals, vitamins and mineral pills alone won't suddenly give you more energy without the food. All of these substances have to work together. Picture these vitamins and minerals as assembly-line workers in a car factory: Just because they show up for work doesn't automatically give you cars off the assembly line; first and foremost, you need the raw materials for them to work with.

That said, you need the B vitamins for energy because they are all essential participants in various metabolic reactions that create, convert or store energy in the body. Here's a brief summary of the various B vitamins and why each is necessary for energy.

Thiamin (vitamin B-1): Works with other B vitamins to convert carbohydrates into usable energy.

Riboflavin (vitamin B-2): Needed to release stored energy for use by the body. Also essential to the function of vitamin B-6 and niacin (vitamin B-3) as a component of several enzymes responsible for the metabolism of carbohydrates, fats, and protein.

Niacin (vitamin B-3): Essential to almost every biochemical link in the metabolism of carbohydrates, protein, and fat for energy.

Pyridoxine (vitamin B-6): Helps convert protein into energy and convert glycogen (the storage form of carbohydrate) into energy for muscle tissue.

Folic acid (folacin): Helps manufacture red blood cells. Specifically, it is required for the synthesis and breakdown of amino acids. Half the women in the U.S. do not consume enough folic acid.

Vitamin B-12: Needed along with folic acid to help manufacture red blood cells. Vitamin B-12 also helps many coenzymes perform their normal metabolic duties.

Pantothenic acid: Helps with the metabolic processing of protein, fat, and carbohydrates.

To see whether or not you are eating at least the recommended daily amounts of the B vitamins, compare your daily food choices to the values listed in Table 6.1. (And recall from the previous chapter that vitamins B-6 and B-12 fall into the category of "vitamins and minerals you need more of as you age." For those two vitamins, your goal should be to consume 150 percent of the RDA.)

Table 6.1. Best Bets For Getting Your B Vitamins

Vitamin	RDA for Adult Women	Food Servings That Provide at Least One-Third the RDA	Amounts Provided
Thiamin (vitamin B-1)	1.1 mg	Beans, cooked from dry (black, lima, navy, pinto, white, lentils, or split peas), 1 cup	0.3–0.4 mg
		Enriched rice, cooked, 1 cup	0.33 mg
		Baked beans, homemade, 1 cup	0.34 mg
		Canadian-style bacon, 2 pieces	0.38 mg
		Roast beef sandwich on bun	0.39 mg
		Acorn squash, baked, 1 cup	0.41 mg
		Peas, cooked from frozen, 1 cup	0.42 mg
		Malt-O-Meal cereal, 1 cup	0.48 mg
		Maypo cereal, ¾ cup	0.50 mg
		Oatmeal, fortified instant, prepared from packet	
		Apple, ¾ cup	0.48 mg
		Maple with raisins, ¾ cup	0.52 mg
		Plain, ¾ cup	0.53 mg
		Bran and cinnamon, ¾ cup	0.56 mg
		Ham, extra lean lunch meat, 2 oz	0.53 mg

(continued next page)

Table 6.1. (continued)

Vitamin	RDA for Adult Women	Food Servings That Provide at Least One-Third the RDA	Amounts Provided
Thiamin (vitamin B-1) (continued)		Pork center rib chop, lean, broiled, braised, or roasted, about 2 oz	0.53–0.66 mg
		Ham, roasted, lean only, 3 oz	0.58 mg
		Pork roast, loin or rib, lean, 3 oz	0.66 mg
		Cheese pizza, thick crust, half of 10" size	0.68 mg
		Pork center loin chop, lean, broiled, braised, or roasted, about 2.5 oz	0.7–0.83 mg
Riboflavin (vitamin B-2)	1.3 mg	2% low-fat milk, 1 cup	0.40 mg
		Fresh raspberry juice, 1 cup	0.40 mg
		Low-fat yogurt, plain or flavored, 1 cup	0.40–0.49 mg
		Macaroni and cheese, homemade, 1 cup	0.40 mg
		1% low-fat milk, 1 cup	0.41 mg
		Mackerel, baked or broiled, 3.5 oz	0.41 mg
		Ham and cheese sandwich	0.41 mg
		Beet greens, cooked, 1 cup	0.42 mg
		Low-fat cottage cheese, 1–2% fat, 1 cup	0.42 mg
		Chicken a la king, 1 cup	0.42 mg
		Spinach, cooked from fresh, 1 cup	0.43 mg
		Ricotta cheese, part skim, 1 cup	0.46 mg
		Soybeans, cooked from dry, 1 cup	0.49 mg
		Soft-serve ice milk, 1 cup	0.54 mg
		Cheese pizza, thick crust, half of 10" size	0.54 mg
		Pacific raw oysters, 1 cup	0.58 mg
		Maypo, ¾ cup	0.60 mg
		Instant oatmeal with bran and raisins, ¾ cup	0.63 mg
		Canned clams, drained, 1 cup	0.68 mg

Table 6.1. (continued)

Vitamin	RDA for Adult Women	Food Servings That Provide at Least One-Third the RDA	Amounts Provided
		Atlantic salmon, canned, small can	0.75 mg
		Canned evaporated skim milk, 1 cup	0.80 mg
Niacin (vitamin B-3)	15 NE (Niacin Equivalents)	Clams, canned, small can	5.4 NE
		Lamb cutlet, lean, cooked, 3 oz	5.4 NE
		Leg of lamb, roasted, lean only, 3 oz	5.4 NE
		Ham sandwich	5.4 NE
		Roast beef sandwich	5.5 NE
		Rabbit, roasted, 3 oz	5.6 NE
		Chicken, dark meat, roasted, 3 oz	5.6 NE
		Venison, roasted, 3 oz	5.7 NE
		Salmon, baked or broiled, 3 oz	5.7 NE
		Malt-O-Meal, 1 cup	5.8 NE
		Turkey, light meat, roasted, 3 oz	5.8 NE
		Peanut butter and jam sandwich	5.8 NE
		Instant oatmeal (average of all flavors), 1 cup	5.9 NE
		Veal, rib, roasted, 3 oz	6.4 NE
		Mackerel, Atlantic, baked or broiled, 3.5 oz	6.9 NE
		Maypo, ¾ cup	7.0 NE
		Veal cutlet, lean, cooked, 3 oz	7.2 NE
		Cheese pizza, thick crust, half of 10″	7.5 NE
		Bluefish, baked or broiled, 3.5 oz	7.8 NE
		Hamburger meat, 4 oz	7.9 NE
		Fresh tuna, baked, 3 oz	9.0 NE
		Sea trout (steelhead), cooked, 3.5 oz	9.7 NE
		Chicken, light meat, roasted, 3 oz	10.6 NE

(continued next page)

Table 6.1. (continued)

Vitamin	RDA for Adult Women	Food Servings That Provide at Least One-Third the RDA	Amounts Provided
Pyridoxine (vitamin B-6)	1.6 mg	Chicken, light meat, roasted, 3 oz	0.52 mg
		Bluefish, baked or broiled, 3.5 oz	0.53 mg
		Prune juice, bottled, 1 cup	0.56 mg
		Canned tuna, light, packed in water, 6-oz can	0.62 mg
		Blue mussels, steamed, meat only, 3 oz	0.63 mg
		Maypo, ¾ cup	0.65 mg
		Banana	0.66 mg
		Chunky turkey soup, ready to serve, 1 cup	0.69 mg
		Baked potato, with skin	0.70 mg
		Tostada with beans and chicken	0.73 mg
		Instant oatmeal (average of all flavors), ¾ cup	0.77 mg
		Sea trout (steelhead), cooked, 3.5 oz	0.80 mg
		Tostada with refried beans	1.00 mg
Folic acid (folacin)	180 µg	Green leaf lettuce, fresh, 1 cup	60 µg
		Artichoke, cooked	61 µg
		Romaine lettuce, fresh, 1 cup	76 µg
		Broccoli, cooked, 1 cup	78 µg
		Garbanzo beans, canned, ½ cup	80 µg
		Dandelion greens, cooked, 1 cup	82 µg
		Turnip greens, cooked, 1 cup	82 µg
		Boysenberries, from frozen, 1 cup	84 µg
		Asparagus, cooked from fresh, ½ cup	88 µg
		Brussels sprouts, cooked, 1 cup	94 µg
		Artichoke hearts, from frozen, 3 oz	95 µg
		Peas, 1 cup	100 µg
		Peanuts, ½ cup	106 µg

Table 6.1. (continued)

Vitamin	RDA for Adult Women	Food Servings That Provide at Least One-Third the RDA	Amounts Provided
		Orange juice, from concentrate, 1 cup	109 µg
		Spinach leaves, fresh, chopped, 1 cup	109 µg
		Black-eyed peas, cooked from frozen, ½ cup	120 µg
		Kidney beans, canned, 1 cup	126 µg
		Collards, cooked from frozen, 1 cup	129 µg
		Sunflower seeds, ½ cup	141 µg
		Lentils, cooked from dry, ½ cup	180 µg
		Spinach, cooked from fresh, 1 cup	262 µg
		Pinto beans, 1 cup	294 µg
Vitamin B-12	2 µg	Instant nonfat dry milk powder, ¼ cup	0.68 µg
		Frozen yogurt (average of all flavors), 1 cup	0.71 µg
		Hamburger meat, 3 oz*	0.78 µg
		Ice milk, regular, 1 cup	0.88 µg
		2% low-fat milk, 1 cup	0.89 µg
		Tuna salad sandwich	0.90 µg
		Skim milk, 1 cup	0.93 µg
		Beef enchilada	1.00 µg
		Cod, baked or broiled, 3.5 oz	1.10 µg
		Low-fat yogurt, fruit, 1 cup	1.10 µg
		Haddock, baked or broiled, 3 oz	1.20 µg
		Ocean perch, baked or broiled, 3.5 oz	1.20 µg
		Northern pike, baked or broiled, 3.5 oz	1.20 µg
		Turkey pastrami, 2 oz	1.20 µg

*In consideration of space, only a select few cuts of beef, and only the most common mixed foods containing beef, are listed.

(continued next page)

Table 6.1. (continued)

Vitamin	RDA for Adult Women	Food Servings That Provide at Least One-Third the RDA	Amounts Provided
Vitamin B-12 (continued)		Turkey sandwich	1.20 µg
		Spaghetti, with meat, 1 cup	1.20 µg
		Turkey ham, 2 oz	1.30 µg
		Low-fat yogurt, plain, 1 cup	1.30 µg
		Beef taco	1.40 µg
		Veal cutlet, broiled, 3 oz	1.40 µg
		Soft-serve ice milk, 1 cup	1.40 µg
		Nonfat yogurt, 1 cup	1.40 µg
		Imitation crab, from surimi, 3 oz	1.40 µg
		Blue mussels, steamed, meat only, 3 oz	1.40 µg
		Carp, baked or broiled, 3.5 oz	1.50 µg
		Shrimp, boiled, 3.5 oz	1.50 µg
		Lasagna with meat, 1 serving	1.50 µg
		Roast beef sandwich	1.50 µg
		Beef and vegetable stew, 1 cup	1.60 µg
		Beef and bean burrito	1.60 µg
		Snapper, baked or broiled, 3.5 oz	1.60 µg
		Sirloin steak, lean only, broiled, 3 oz	1.70 µg
		Tostada with beef and beans	1.70 µg
		Extra-lean ground beef, broiled or fried, 3 oz	1.80 µg
		Tuna noodle casserole, 1 cup	1.80 µg
		Meatloaf, beef only, 1 serving	1.90 µg
		Scallops, steamed, 3.5 oz	1.90 µg
		Catfish, fried in cornmeal, 3.5 oz	2.00 µg
		Sole, baked or broiled, 3 oz	2.10 µg
		Lamb cutlet, cooked, 3 oz	2.20 µg
		Round steak, lean only, broiled, 3 oz	2.50 µg
		Pollock, baked or broiled, 3.5 oz	3.10 µg
		Rockfish, baked or broiled, 3.5 oz	3.20 µg
		Bass, baked or broiled, 3.5 oz	3.40 µg

Table 6.1. (continued)

Vitamin	RDA for Adult Women	Food Servings That Provide at Least One-Third the RDA	Amounts Provided
		Lobster, cooked, meat only, 1 cup	4.50 µg
		Salmon, baked or broiled, 3 oz	4.90 µg
		Canned tuna, light, packed in water, 6-oz can	5.60 µg
		Bluefish, baked or broiled, 3.5 oz	7.10 µg
		Manhattan-style clam chowder, 1 cup	7.90 µg
		Sardines, canned, 3.5 oz	9.00 µg
		Fresh crab, blue or Dungeness, 1 cup	10.00 µg
		Herring, baked or broiled, 3.5 oz	13.00 µg
		Mackerel, Atlantic, baked or broiled, 3.5 oz	19.00 µg
		Raw oysters, 1 cup	40.00– 48.00 µg
		Steamed clams, meat only, about 20	89.00 µg
		Clams, canned, 1 cup	158.00 µg
Pantothenic acid*	There is no RDA but 4–7 mg is generally considered safe and adequate	Hubbard squash, baked, 1 cup	1.00 mg
		Soft-serve ice milk, 1 cup	1.00 mg
		Chicken, dark meat, roasted, 3 oz	1.00 mg
		Mashed potatoes with milk, 1 cup	1.00 mg
		Veal cutlet, lean, cooked, 3 oz	1.10 mg
		Green peas, cooked from fresh, 1 cup	1.10 mg
		Split peas, cooked from dry, 1 cup	1.20 mg
		Baked potato, with skin	1.20 mg
		Low-fat yogurt, plain and flavored, 1 cup	1.20 mg
		Trout, baked or broiled, 3 oz	1.20 mg
		Acorn squash, baked, 1 cup	1.20 mg
		Duck, roasted, meat only, 3 oz	1.30 mg

*In order to include more items, foods with at least one-quarter of the RDA are listed for pantothenic acid.

(continued next page)

Table 6.1.   (continued)

Vitamin	RDA for Adult Women	Food Servings That Provide at Least One-Third the RDA	Amounts Provided
Pantothenic acid (continued)		Frozen yogurt (average of all flavors), 1 cup	1.30 mg
		Nonfat yogurt, 1 cup	1.50 mg
		Turkey, dark meat, roasted, 3 oz	1.50 mg
		Mushrooms, cooked, ½ cup	1.70 mg
		Evaporated skim milk, 1 cup	1.80 mg
		Sea trout (steelhead), 3.5 oz	2.25 mg
		Chili with beans, canned, 1 cup	3.60 mg

HOW TO SPEED UP YOUR CALORIE BURNERS

Here's the bad news. Through menopause and thereafter your body fat percentage generally increases while your lean body mass (muscle tissue) generally decreases. All this results in a gradual decline in your basal metabolic rate, which is the amount of calories your body requires just to maintain minimal functioning of your body (body temperature, heart rate, breathing, and so on). Thus, if you didn't change anything—the amount and kinds of food you eat or your level of physical activity—you'd be likely to gain weight slowly during and after menopause. Why? Because you'd be eating the same number of calories but your body would be burning fewer.

This decline in metabolism is the reason menopausal women must eat fewer calories each day to maintain their weight. However, just cutting calories isn't the answer, because many of our nutrient needs have increased—for calcium, vitamin D, and antioxidants, not to mention nutrients like vitamin B-12 and zinc that aren't fully absorbed as we grow older. So if you simply cut down on food, you'd lose out on essential nutrition.

What's the answer? Don't take this lying down—literally. There are ways of raising your metabolic rate, and they work even in your fifties, sixties, and beyond.

Burn More Calories with a High-Carbohydrate Diet

You can burn more calories simply by eating foods high in carbohydrates instead of fat. For your body uses more energy (burns more calories) to metabolize carbohydrates than it does to break down food fat and store it as body fat. For example, if you eat 100 high-fat calories of peanut butter and your body doesn't use the calories for energy right at the moment, 97 of the 100 calories will, most likely, end up being deposited in fat tissue. But if you eat 100 low-fat calories of bread above and beyond your energy needs, only 77 calories will be deposited as fat because your body will burn 23 calories to digest, convert, and store those mostly carbohydrate calories.

One recent study concluded that the human body has several hormonal systems in place to help handle the bigger influxes of carbohydrate and protein calories. But as far as we know, the body does not have any such system for fat.

Eat Small, Frequent Meals

You can even use the digestive process in your own body to help burn more calories while you're at rest. Each time you eat, you set your body's digestive process in motion, and this startup burns calories. So the more frequently you eat, the more calories you can burn just in digesting your food. This strategy works as long as you're not eating more calories, but just eating the same number spaced across several smaller meals.

Build Muscle Power

Muscle cells burn more calories at rest than fat cells do. So the more muscle you have, the more energy you burn even while resting. Approximately 70 percent of the calories you burn in a day are due to the metabolic activity of lean body mass (muscle). If you work to build your lean body mass, you can counteract the decrease in total calories burned each day that we see in women after menopause. But how do you make more muscles? Should you eat high-protein foods or drink high-priced protein powders? No. The only way to build muscle is to *use* muscle. If you want to gain muscle weight instead of fat tissue, *exercise* has to be part of the equation. And for the best results, you should do a combination of aerobic conditioning and strength training.

Aerobic Conditioning

If the only way to build muscle is to use muscle, then any exercise that uses some muscle—like walking, gardening, golf, tennis, or bicycling—will have a positive impact on at least maintaining and possibly building muscle. **Aerobic exercise,** sustained, vigorous activities that allow oxygen from the lungs to get to working muscles, will have the added benefit of strengthening your lung and cardiac capacity. Good examples of aerobic exercise are swimming, power walking, aerobics classes, or using home exercise equipment such as rowing machines, stationary bicycles, or treadmills with arm movement (and where you are the motor driving the floor belt).

Strength Training

Performing strength-training exercises only two or three times a week will help boost your muscle mass. And you don't have to become a bodybuilder or bench-press your weight to benefit from strength training. Anyone can build muscles through appropriate exercises. Other words for strength training are resistance training, weight training, and isotonics. Whatever the name, strength-training exercises usually involve activities that you repeat 8 to 12 times in a row while standing or sitting in one place. Some examples are leg lifts (you may have to do more than 12 to reach the point of exhaustion, though), weightlifting, and arm curls. These exercises push a muscle (or set of muscles) to exhaustion, which encourages the muscle to grow and improve its tone. Strength training can be done two to three times a week for 30 to 40 minutes each session.

Here are six good reasons to start strength training today:

1. It builds muscle mass and keeps you active and stronger for daily activities. You may even find yourself walking faster or carrying heavy burdens more easily than before.
2. It raises your body's metabolic rate since muscle mass requires more calories to sustain itself than body fat does.
3. It increases bone density, thereby helping reduce the risk of osteoporosis.
4. It decreases the risk for developing diabetes in later years. The more muscle mass you have, the less insulin is required to get sugar from the blood to body tissues. Enough muscle makes it more likely that your body will have enough insulin.
5. It can improve the ratio of your HDL ("good") cholesterol to your LDL ("bad") cholesterol, possibly helping to reduce the risk for heart disease.
6. It eases the pain of osteoarthritis and may even ease the pain of rheumatoid arthritis.

Exercise Regularly

Simply exercising burns extra calories, of course. But recent research although still considered controversial, has suggested that you burn calories a faster rate for even 4 to 12 hours *after* exercise, thus helping to raise your basal metabolic rate. And beginners benefit the most: The less trained you are, the longer your metabolism stays elevated.

If you stick with a regular exercise program though, there are even greater rewards waiting for you. After exercising aerobically for about 20 minutes, the experienced exerciser is probably primarily burning fat for fuel.

(Beginners tend to use glucose as their main fuel during aerobic exercise. But once you get into a regular exercise program and become more fit, your body will shift to burning fat.) Aerobic activities include walking, swimming, biking, aerobic dance, and rowing. Most experts recommend aerobic workouts lasting 30 to 40 minutes several times a week. However, if you don't have a 30-minute chunk of free time during your day, you can still profit from pacing your aerobic workout through your day in shifts. Thus, you could have a 10-minute stationary bike ride in the morning, a 10-minute walk at lunch, and a 10-minute treadmill jog before or after dinner. The health and weight-loss benefits may not match those provided by a solid 30-minute workout, but they are far better than if you'd done nothing. Indeed, try incorporating as many brief moments of physical activity as you can into your day. It's as easy as:

- Taking the stairs instead of elevators.
- Walking to nearby destinations instead of taking the car.
- Jumping on the treadmill or stationary bike during a 10-minute phone conversation instead of sitting or standing.
- Getting out of your chair more often at work.
- Getting up to change the TV channel instead of using the remote control (or better yet, spend less time watching TV).
- Parking farther away from your destination and walking the rest of the way.

Research on exercise is constantly providing us with new information, so be sure to consult your doctor before beginning a new exercise program and for the latest expert advice.

HOW TO EAT FOR MORE ENERGY

We've covered a lot of material in this chapter, so let's recap the important points.

There are four main ways to eat for more energy:

1. Keep your body fueled with energy, by eating the right *type* of calories: lowfat meals with some protein but mostly carbohydrates.
2. Make these calories hit your bloodstream at the right *times*: Eat small, frequent meals throughout the day, and eat light at night.
3. Make sure you get the RDA for iron, zinc, and vitamins A, C, and E, all of which nutrients play essential roles in metabolic processes.
4. Make sure you get at least the RDA for all the B vitamins—and, actually, 150 percent of the RDA for vitamins B-6 and B-12 (recall Diet Commandment #4).

The next section of the book—Part Three, consisting of chapters 7 and 8—discusses how to prevent osteoporosis, cancer, and heart disease by developing good nutritional habits. The second five Diet Commandments will be presented in this section.

PART THREE

HOW DIET CAN HELP PREVENT DISEASE

7

A STRONG DIET FOR STRONG BONES: PREVENTING OSTEOPOROSIS

*O*steoporosis. It's a word that can send shivers down your spine. Maybe you've had a relative who battled hip or spinal fractures in older age, or perhaps you remember an aunt or grandmother with a slumped-over back.

Until about age 30 or 35, your body was building your bones, adding more calcium and other minerals to make them stronger. Up through those years, the object of the game was to build as much bone mass as possible. By the time you start thinking about menopause, however, you're past that point. Your total bone mass has started gradually declining. But all is not lost. For although you can't build more bone mass, you can *preserve* the bone mass you have.

ARE YOU AT RISK FOR OSTEOPOROSIS?

For many older adults, including about one-third of postmenopausal women, bone loss accelerates too quickly, a condition known as **osteoporosis.** In osteoporosis, the protein matrix of bone and the mineral deposits are gradually lost, decreasing the total amount of bone and weakening the skeleton. These weakened bones are then more susceptible to fractures. Osteoporotic fractures occur primarily in the hips, spine, and wrists.

At least 15 to 20 million people in the United States have osteoporosis. Whites, postmenopausal women, and older adults in general are most at risk. Though genetic factors play some part, according to some bone metabolism experts, fully half of your bone loss after age 30 (when your peak bone mass is reached) is influenced by lifestyle factors. Fortunately, you can control most of these to some extent.

To assess your own risk for developing osteoporosis, answer the questions below.

	Circle One	
Are you a woman?	Yes	No
Are you White or Asian?	Yes	No
Do you have a family history of osteoporosis?	Yes	No
Do you have a small body frame?	Yes	No
Have you been underweight during a portion of your adult life?	Yes	No
Did you start menstruating later than most girls your age?	Yes	No
Have you stopped menstruating?	Yes	No
Did you bear no children during your adult years?	Yes	No
Did you have a complete hysterectomy?	Yes	No
Did you go through menopause earlier than the average woman?	Yes	No
Do you smoke?	Yes	No
Do you drink substantial amounts of alcohol (more than two drinks a day)?	Yes	No
Would you describe yourself as sedentary or, at the other end of the spectrum, as one who has exercised excessively during her adult life?	Yes	No
Were calcium-rich foods, like dairy products, largely missing from your diet between the ages of 15 and 30?	Yes	No

The more "Yes" answers you have, the higher your risk of developing osteoporosis. This means that the dietary and other lifestyle suggestions given in this chapter are especially important for you. You'll also want to answer the questions below, to assess whether (or to what degree) your current diet is adding to your risk of developing osteoporosis—although you may have difficulty answering some items before you read the discussion on diet that follows.

	Circle One	
Are you consuming less than the RDA of calcium (800–1,500 mg)?	Yes	No
Are you consuming less than the RDA of vitamin D (200 IU), and do you rarely spend time outdoors and in the sun?	Yes	No

Are you getting none of your calcium with lactose, found in milk and some milk products?	Yes	No
Are you consuming less than the RDA of magnesium (280 mg)?	Yes	No
Do you tend to eat twice the RDA of protein (the RDA of protein is 46 grams for the 58-kilogram or 128-pound woman)?	Yes	No
Do you tend to drink more than a couple cups of coffee (or other caffeinated beverages) every day?	Yes	No
Do you tend to drink an excessive amount of alcohol (more than two drinks a day)?	Yes	No
Do you tend to consume less than the RDA for calcium and drink several carbonated soft drinks a day?	Yes	No
Do you tend to eat a very high-fiber diet (about 40 g of fiber or more every day)?	Yes	No

The more "Yes" answers you have, the more your diet is adding to your risk of developing osteoporosis.

BONE BOOSTERS

Scientists do not currently know of either a surefire cure for or a completely proven preventive strategy to avoid developing osteoporosis. They do, however, recommend some dietary and lifestyle practices that seem to be associated with decreasing the likelihood of osteoporosis and possibly slowing the natural bone loss that tends to accompany old age. In fact, you can figure out most of their recommendations by reviewing the questions you just answered. While you obviously can't change your gender, race, or past diet history, you can correct any current lifestyle and dietary habits to which you answered "Yes." Here are the types of actions to consider.

Exercise

Probably the best thing you can do for your bones is to engage in weight-bearing exercise. Try walking, aerobics, using a treadmill, playing tennis, or any other exercise where you're putting your body weight on your feet and then shifting it. You can reduce bone loss by getting 45 to 60 minutes of such weight-bearing exercise four times a week. Remember, though, that only weight-bearing exercise, not swimming or bicycling, directly benefits bone mass. That isn't to say that exercises like swimming or bicycling don't benefit your body in other ways (such as aerobic conditioning and enhancing flexibility), but simply that they're not going to help preserve bone mass as effectively as the other types of exercise.

Hormone Replacement Therapy

As we have discussed, HRT adds estrogen and progesterone hormones back into your body, thereby helping reduce the rate of bone loss and your risk of osteoporosis. The estrogen is essentially convincing your body that you are neither going through nor have gone through menopause. But HRT also brings its own possible risks (for estrogen-dependent cancers) and unpleasant side effects. For more information on the risks and benefits of HRT, see chapter 2.

Diet

A good osteoporosis-fighting diet is more complicated than drinking a couple of glasses of milk—although that's certainly a great start. The rest of this chapter will help you understand why so many dietary factors contribute to bone health during menopause and beyond. But remember that researchers do caution us not to take any of these dietary or lifestyle approaches to the extreme. Getting too much exercise or consuming too much calcium or vitamin D can be harmful. More is not always better.

Finally, if you are at high risk for osteoporosis, you might want to discuss other approaches with your doctor. Experimental treatments include **calcitonin injections** (a calcium-regulating hormone approved by the FDA for treating osteoporosis), **etidronate** (a drug used to treat other diseases; not yet approved for use with osteoporosis, but has been shown to restore bone and prevent fracture in some cases), and **fluoride** (the ionized form of fluorine used by your body), among others.

THE HEALTHY-BONE DIET

To keep your bones as healthy as possible, you need to focus on three main dietary goals: getting enough calcium, getting enough calcium-absorption enhancers so you can use more of the calcium you do consume, and avoiding calcium depleters that rob you of valuable calcium.

Getting Enough Calcium

Most people become concerned about calcium when the threat of osteoporosis starts looming in their not-so-distant future—or when they break a bone. Calcium is probably the first nutrient that comes to mind when we think of osteoporosis, and justifiably so. However, since your body uses calcium to build bone only until you're 30 or 35, why do you still need to keep up your calcium intake when you're 50 or 60? We often think of the human skeleton as tough and permanent, but our bone is actually living tissue. Whenever the amount of calcium in our diet is less than what our body needs, the body can make up the difference by withdrawing calcium from our body's best calcium bank account, the bones. The bones make this sacrifice because calcium also helps muscles contract, including the all-important heart muscle. Calcium is also part of other life-sustaining processes such as blood clotting, nerve cell transmission and enzyme activity. In other words, we need calcium for several vital body functions, and we don't want to be overdrawn at the bone bank to get the calcium we need.

The majority of research data (though not all studies) does suggest that calcium intake might help decrease bone loss in postmenopausal women. Research suggests postmenopausal women can decrease bone loss as much as 50 percent by getting enough calcium daily. Women taking estrogen pills apparently reap those same benefits with a bit less calcium. And even if the high amounts of calcium intake have only a slight effect on bone loss, a little more bone goes a long way. *The Proceedings of the Society for Experimental Biology and Medicine* reports that even small increases in bone mass can actually cut fracture rates by quite a bit.

How Much Calcium Is Enough?

Recently the National Institutes of Health appointed a Consensus Development Panel on Optimal Calcium Intake. And this panel recommended that postmenopausal women between 50 and 64 who are not on estrogen or hormone replacement therapy, and all women over 65, consume 1,500 milligrams of calcium a day. The panel also recommended about 1,000 milligrams a day for postmenopausal women currently taking estrogen.

However, most women fall short of the current RDA of 800 milligrams of calcium, let alone this higher standard. Indeed, most American women get barely half the RDA. What kind of advice do experts offer American women who don't get enough calcium? There are two main points:

1. Get as much calcium as you can from food, using calcium supplements only to fill in the gaps. (If you have had calcium-containing kidney stones, you should check first with your physician on this and other calcium advice.)
2. Supplementation much higher than the RDA is *not* recommended, mainly because excessive calcium can interfere with the absorption of other important minerals like iron and zinc and with the effectiveness of certain medications.

This brings us to another Diet Commandment.

DIET COMMANDMENT #6

Eat at Least Two Calcium-Rich Foods Every Day,
Preferably Ones Also High in Vitamin D

What If You're Not a Milk Drinker?
Can you realistically get 1,000 to 1,500 milligrams of calcium from your diet
if you're not a milk drinker? As a matter of fact, you can.

It's difficult—but not impossible. Here's how:

- Drink just one glass of nonfat or low-fat milk as a between-meal beverage. (A little chocolate syrup turns a glass of plain milk into a chocolate
  treat.) You get a good dose of calcium (316 mg) along with lactose, vitamin D, and a little bit of magnesium, all of which are calcium-absorption
  enhancers.
- Take a vitamin-mineral supplement that contains 100 percent of the
  RDA for vitamin D and some calcium (15 to 25 percent of the RDA, or
  about 200 mg).
- Eat a leafy green vegetable or a bean dish every day. (We should do this
  anyway, for other health benefits.) One cup of broccoli, for example,
  provides 180 milligrams of calcium.
- Choose one item each day from the calcium "high rollers," a list that includes yogurt, hot cocoa, cheese pizza, low-fat frozen yogurt, and many
  other tasty foods. One cup of low-fat flavored yogurt, for example, provides 345 milligrams of calcium.

Add these items together, and you get around 1,050 milligrams!

Food Sources of Calcium
There are basically two types of calcium-rich foods, those from plants and
those from cows. Do you need to eat dairy foods to get enough calcium?
Well, yes and no. Theoretically, you *can* get from 1,000 to 1,500 milligrams
of calcium from plant foods alone—but, as the above discussion demon-
strates, it isn't easy. Drinking just a little nonfat or low-fat milk every day is
certainly going to help the cause. Eating a carton of low-fat yogurt or a couple of ounces of reduced-fat cheese will further improve your calcium intake. See Table 7.1 for a listing of the foods highest in calcium, including a
subcategory of beans and vegetables high in calcium.

Calcium through Food or Supplements?

Several controlled clinical trials have demonstrated significant reduction in the rate of bone loss in postmenopausal women who took calcium supplements. In one study, normal postmenopausal women who consumed about 750 milligrams of calcium from food (a fairly typical amount), were given an additional 1,000 milligrams of calcium in a supplement. The bone loss in their axial and appendicular bones (trunk and extremities) significantly slowed. On the other hand, the *New England Journal of Medicine* reported on a study that showed that, if you usually consume less than 400 milligrams of calcium, increasing your daily intake to 800 milligrams *through food alone* can also reduce bone loss.

If you are considering taking a calcium supplement, you should first ask yourself if you are already getting the recommended daily amount of calcium for women over 50 (1,000 to 1,500 mg) in your normal diet. Because if you are, extra calcium from supplements probably isn't going to do you any extra good. Recent studies have shown that calcium supplements weren't helpful for women who already met their requirement for calcium. (Chapter 10 will help you determine how much calcium you're currently getting in your diet.)

Moreover, one national expert, Janet King, Ph.D., a registered dietitian, believes it is better to get your calcium from food. Dr. King sees a real risk in taking calcium supplements totaling 500 to 1,000 milligrams a day, because the amount of calcium in most of these supplements is much greater than the amount you get in a food source. The salt form of calcium from supplements may bind with other minerals more than calcium in regular food does. Calcium supplements can also interfere with the absorption of certain medications, such as tetracycline. So if you are taking any medications, be sure to consult your doctor or nurse practitioner *before* taking any calcium supplement.

How to Get the Best Results with Calcium Supplements

If you are going to take calcium supplements, here are some suggestions on how to get the best results.

- *Take the absorption test* to find out if your calcium supplement is useful. To do the test, drop your calcium tablet in half a cup of plain vinegar. After 30 minutes, check the cup. If your tablet has disintegrated, it will dissolve in your stomach and be available for absorption. If your tablet has *not* completely disintegrated, you probably aren't getting the amount of calcium from your supplement that you think you're getting. You may want to consider another brand.

Table 7.1. Calcium High Rollers

Food	Calcium (mg)	Calories	Fat (g)
Best Bets			
Yogurt, plain, nonfat, 1 cup	451	126	0.4
Yogurt, plain, low-fat, 1 cup	414	143	3.5
Instant breakfast drink, made with nonfat milk, 12 oz	376	261	0.5
Yogurt, nonfat, sugar-free with fruit, 1 cup	369	122	0.4
Parmesan cheese, shredded, 1 oz	355	129	7.7
Nonfat dry milk powder, 1 oz	349	101	0.2
Yogurt, low-fat, flavored, 1 cup	345	231	2.5
Oatmeal, homemade (½ cup oats with 1 cup 1% low-fat milk)	333	260	5.0
Alba, sugar-free cocoa mix plus calcium, 1 packet	327	62	0.5
Milk, nonfat, 1 cup	316	90	0.6
Milk, 1% low-fat, 1 cup	312	104	2.4
Low-fat frozen yogurt, 1 cup	300	202	4.0
Milk, 2% low-fat, 1 cup	296	121	5.0
Milk, whole (3.3% fat), 1 cup	291	149	8.0
Buttermilk, 8 oz	284	92	2.0
Spinach, boiled and drained, 1 cup	277	53	0.4
Swiss cheese, low-fat, 1 oz	272	51	2.0
Tofu, firm, ½ cup	258	181	11.0
Cheese pizza, 1 slice	220	290	9.0
Premium ice milk, 1 cup	216	242	8.0
Sugar-free cocoa mix, unfortified, small packet	213	48	0.5
Mozzarella cheese, part-skim (low-moisture), 1 oz	207	79	5.0
Sockeye salmon, canned, 3 oz	203	130	6.0
Macaroni and cheese, 1 cup	200	230	10.0
Low-fat processed American cheese, 1 oz	194	51	2.0
Evaporated skim milk, ¼ cup	184	50	0.0
Pink salmon with bones, canned, 3 oz	181	118	5.0
Collard greens, boiled from frozen, ½ cup	179	31	0.3

Table 7.1. (continued)

Food	Calcium (mg)	Calories	Fat (g)
Waffle, from mix	179	206	8.0*
Ricotta cheese, part-skim, 1/4 cup	167	85	5.0
Instant oatmeal, fortified, 1 packet	160	105	4.0
Good Bets			
Vanilla pudding, made with 2% low-fat milk, 1/2 cup	146	144	2.4
Scalloped potatoes, from recipe, 1 cup	140	210	9.0
Blackstrap molasses, 1 Tbsp	136	43	0.0
Fudgsicle bar	129	91	0.2
Ocean perch, baked or broiled, 3 oz	117	103	1.8
Hot chocolate or cocoa, 1 packet	92	102	1.0
Clams, steamed, boiled, or canned, 3 oz	78	125	1.7
Low-fat cottage cheese, 1/2 cup	77	82	2.0
Freshwater bass, baked or broiled, 3 oz	73	106	3.4
Rainbow trout, baked or broiled, 3 oz	73	128	5.0
Cream of wheat or Maypo, 1/2 cup	62	85	1.2
Shrimp, medium, baked or broiled, 3 oz	55	132	4.4
Pacific halibut, steamed, 3 oz	51	111	2.5
Dungeness crab, steamed, 3 oz	50	86	1.0
Good Bets for Vegetarians			
Spinach, boiled from frozen, 1/2 cup	139	27	0.2
Turnip greens, boiled, 1/2 cup	124	25	0.3
Broccoli, cooked from frozen, 1 cup	94	52	0.2
Kale, boiled from frozen, 1/2 cup	90	20	0.3
Beet greens, boiled, 1/2 cup	82	20	0.1
Bok choy, boiled, 1/2 cup	79	10	0.1
Baked beans, homemade, 1/2 cup	77	190	6.5
Dandelion greens, cooked, 1/2 cup	74	17	0.3
Small white beans, boiled, 1/2 cup	65	127	0.6
Navy beans, boiled, 1/2 cup	64	129	0.5
Great northern beans, boiled, 1/2 cup	60	104	0.4
Red kidney beans, boiled, 1/2 cup	58	109	0.1
Fresh spinach leaves, chopped, 1 cup	56	25	0.2

*The fat can be reduced by using a "light" mix or adding less oil than the mix directions call for.

•   *Use a supplement with calcium carbonate.* These contain the greatest amount of calcium per tablet, so you will need to take fewer tablets. Reducing the number of tablets is useful if you must get almost all your calcium from supplements (if, for instance, you're severely lactose-intolerant).

•   *Take your multivitamin with iron at a different time* than your extra calcium supplement. Calcium supplements can inhibit iron absorption.

•   *Take calcium supplements before bedtime.* According to some evidence, that may be the best time. Although between meals, during the day, is probably also effective.

•   *Take your calcium supplement with lots of water* to discourage constipation.

•   *Do not take calcium supplements around the time you take bulk-forming laxatives,* because this may reduce your absorption of the calcium.

•   *Avoid calcium supplements from "natural" sources* such as bonemeal, crushed oyster shell, or dolomite. "Natural" may sound good, but these supplements may have dangerously high levels of toxic minerals like lead and other toxic metals.

Don't Take Too Much Calcium

Don't exceed 1,500 milligrams of calcium a day from all sources. Too much calcium can interfere with the absorption of other minerals, cause constipation, and increase your risk of urinary stone formation and kidney dysfunction. Some experts consider 2,500 milligrams of calcium safe for adults, unless there is a personal or family history of kidney problems. However, even if you have no history of kidney problems, try to limit your total intake of calcium, from food and any supplements you may take, to 1,500 milligrams daily.

If you are already on hormone or estrogen replacement therapy expressly to help prevent osteoporosis, or if you are thinking about going on it, taking calcium supplements may allow you to take half the usual dose of estrogen, thereby reducing the risks and side effects of HRT. Researchers have found that postmenopausal women taking a combination of 1,000 milligrams of calcium and half the usual dose of estrogen experience the same bone mass maintenance benefits as the women taking estrogen at the full dose with no calcium supplement.

Getting Enough Calcium-Absorption Enhancers

Normally, a person's intestines can absorb only 30 to 50 percent of the calcium eaten. Thus, the actual amount your system absorbs might be substantially less than the amount you consume. Fortunately, certain food components help your body absorb more calcium from food. So, to keep your

Table 7.2. Foods That Help You Absorb Calcium

Calcium-Absorption Enhancers	Food Sources
Vitamin D	Milks that are fortified with vitamin D, egg yolks, products made with fortified milk
Lactose	All milks and some milk products, including ice cream, yogurt, and cottage cheese
Magnesium	Nuts and legumes; certain leafy green vegetables, such as broccoli and spinach; potatoes; and, to a lesser extent, whole-grain foods, meats, seafood, and milk
Boron	Generally speaking, fruits, vegetables, tubers, and legumes have the highest concentrations of boron

calcium levels high, include in your diet foods with these calcium-absorption enhancers: lactose, vitamin D, and magnesium (see Table 7.2), and also boron (see chapter 4). These components are often found in foods already rich in calcium, such as milk, milk products, and green vegetables.

This absorption enhancing ability is another reason to get as much calcium as possible from food sources rather than to rely completely on supplements. Interestingly, another calcium-absorption enhancer is stomach acid, the hydrochloric acid released after you eat a meal or snack to help start digestion.

If You're Lactose-Intolerant

Lactose intolerance is a partial or complete inability to digest **lactose,** the primary sugar in milk. Lactose must be broken down before it can be absorbed. This is done by the enzyme **lactase,** which under normal circumstances is conveniently produced in the intestine. But production of lactase can go awry due to genetics, age, and gastrointestinal distress or malnutrition. People who are lactose-intolerant suffer from diarrhea, bloating, gas, and nausea after drinking milk or eating dairy products.

There are varying degrees of lactose intolerance, too. Some people can consume low-lactose dairy products without discomfort; others can't. For your information, Table 7.3 lists various dairy products and the amounts of lactose in a typical serving of each. You are the best judge of how much lactose your system can comfortably tolerate.

Fortunately, there are ways for lactose-intolerant people to get their calcium without triggering problems. They can:

- Eat smaller servings of dairy products several times a day instead of one large serving.
- Eat dairy products with a meal or in a recipe with other ingredients to dilute the concentration of lactose.
- Eat aged natural cheeses (like cheddar) because they tend to have less lactose than other cheeses due to the production and aging processes.
- Eat fermented milk products (like yogurt) that contain bacterial enzymes that break down some of the lactose.
- Use lactose-reduced milk as a beverage or in cooking, or add lactase enzyme products to milk to help break down some of the lactose.
- Beef up your diet with vegetable and other nondairy sources of calcium, like tofu, spinach, blackstrap molasses, greens, broccoli, and several kinds of beans (see Table 7.1).

For a list of the best plant sources of calcium, see the discussion of Diet Commandment #6 in chapter 9.

Vitamin D and Calcium—A Winning Combination

Vitamin D is a doubly good friend to calcium because it helps increase the amount of calcium retained by the kidneys (which means you lose less calcium through urine), and it also increases the amount of calcium absorbed from food in the intestinal tract. In fact, without enough vitamin D, calcium cannot be absorbed at all. But the two together are a winning combination. One recent study, reported in the *New England Journal of Medicine,* supplemented the diets of over 1,600 elderly women with 1,200 milligrams of calcium and 800 IU of vitamin D for 18 months. The bone density of the proximal femur (thigh bone) actually increased by an average of 2.7 percent. What happened to the women in the study who were *not* given the calcium and vitamin D? Their thigh bone density decreased by an average of 4.6 percent.

Table 7.3. How Much Lactose Do Dairy Foods Contain?

Dairy Food	Lactose Content (g)
Cow's milk (with milk solids added), 1 cup	14
Cow's milk (with no solids added), 1 cup	12
Buttermilk, 1 cup	12
Yogurt, 1 cup	9
Ice cream, 1 cup	8
Cottage cheese, 1 cup	6
Cheddar cheese, 2 oz	Trace

The RDA for vitamin D is 200 IU This amount is easy to get if you drink fortified milk every day or eat foods made with lots of fortified milk. If you can tolerate milk well, it may be a good idea to drink a glass of vitamin D–enriched nonfat or low-fat milk as a snack, between-meal beverage, or with a meal once every day.

Also, the body can make enough vitamin D on its own when the skin is exposed to good old-fashioned sunshine. (Ultraviolet light changes a compound in the skin, **7-dehydrocholesterol,** into vitamin D.) But your skin starts making less and less of it as you age. An 80-year-old's skin has half the ability to make vitamin D as that of a 20-year-old. Probably those Americans most at risk of not making enough vitamin D are those living in the northern United States, especially during the winter months, and older people in general, especially those confined to their homes or institutionalized. Try to expose at least your face and hands to the sun for at least 30 minutes each day, especially in winter months. Use a lotion with a sun protection factor (SPF) of 4 or 6 for shorter exposures to sunlight; this level of protection will minimize damage from the sun while letting enough rays in to promote some production of vitamin D in the skin.

If you decide to take a vitamin-mineral supplement, make sure it contains not much more than the RDA for vitamin D (200 IU). For vitamin D can be toxic in daily doses of 1,000 IU or more. Investigative studies are currently going on to find out more about the role vitamin D plays in not only osteoporosis prevention but also cardiovascular function, blood pressure, diabetes mellitus, cancer, and the immune system.

Magnesium and Boron

Magnesium increases calcium absorption from the intestines and helps the body use vitamin D. It also plays a role in maintaining the completeness of bone. Boron works a bit differently from other calcium-absorption enhancers. Instead of enhancing calcium absorption from the small intestines, like lactose and magnesium, it may discourage the loss of calcium through the urine. Recent evidence suggests that diets deficient in boron (and diets low in fruits and vegetables are usually low in boron) can cause you to lose too much calcium through the urine.

Avoiding Calcium Depleters

Your body can lose more calcium than it needs to in two ways: (1) via the kidneys when calcium is pulled from the bloodstream and released in urine, and (2) via the intestinal tract when less calcium is absorbed from food by the intestinal wall.

Here are the foods or food components that can make you lose calcium via the kidneys.

• *Animal protein.* Animal protein increases the amount of calcium you lose through your urine. Some researchers hypothesize that lowering the animal protein in your diet may actually reduce the amount of calcium needed in the diet.

• *Caffeine.* Researchers at the University of San Diego examined the relationship between caffeine intake and bone density in 980 postmenopausal women and found that a glass of milk a day kept the negative effects of caffeine away. The women who drank at least one glass of milk a day showed *no* relationship between caffeine and bone density, while the women who did not consume milk but did consume caffeine showed some loss of bone density.

So, what's a coffee lover to do? Limit your consumption of coffee of any kind to no more than two cups a day. (Keeping the lid on coffee will provide other health benefits as well, because all coffee contains tannins that may inhibit the absorption of some minerals.) Another suggestion for those of you who love coffee but hate drinking milk as a beverage: Try ordering a double decaf latte with nonfat milk. This way you can get your milk for the day and satisfy your morning coffee craving with minimal caffeine.

These are the foods or food components that can make you absorb less calcium via the intestinal tract.

• *Alcohol.* Excessive alcohol can inhibit calcium absorption. Alcohol also reduces the amount of active vitamin D formed by the body and may interfere with the bone-protecting benefits of estrogen. Alcohol may even increase the loss of calcium via the kidneys.

• *Phosphorus.* Phosphorus competes with calcium for absorption in the intestines. Many foods that contain phosphorus—like milk, milk products, and meats—pose no problem. However, avoid dietary extras like soda and beer that contain phosphorus and do not contribute any other required nutrients. A study reported in the *Journal of Orthopedic Research* showed that women who drank carbonated beverages had 2.3 times as great a rate of bone fractures after age 40 as those who didn't drink soda. The researchers even found a significant relationship between the *amount* of soda and the *number* of fractures in women over age 40.

Especially after age 50, it's a good idea to limit your soda consumption to one or two a day, if at all. What your body really needs most—what it's thirsting for more than anything else—is *water.*

• *Fiber/phytates.* Phytates are a kind of phosphorus that contain organic compounds, which, when present in the intestines, decrease the amount of minerals absorbed. Fiber and phytates can bind with calcium in the intestinal tract so that calcium is simply unable to be absorbed. Whole grains, bran, and some soy products contain phytates and are also high in fiber.

• *Oxalates.* Oxalates are organic acids that can merge with calcium in the intestinal tract to form complexes that cannot dissolve in water and therefore cannot be easily absorbed. Oxalates are primarily found in spinach, rhubarb, and chocolate.

Of course, fiber/phytates and oxalates are all substances found in foods, such as whole grains and leafy green vegetables, that we need for other vital nutrients. So it doesn't make much sense to curtail our consumption of these foods. However, it does make sense to limit our consumption of the other calcium depleters, animal protein, caffeine, alcohol, and soft drinks. Remember Diet Commandment #3: Limit your intake of caffeine, soft drinks, and alcohol—and drink plenty of water.

Why Limit Your Intake of Caffeine?

Caffeine is a stimulant—and it stimulates more than just your brain. Doses at the level of 3 to 5 mg/kg/day (for a 150-pound person, this would be 204 to 341 mg, or the amount contained in two to four cups of regular coffee, depending on its strength) can produce mild anxiety, cardiovascular effects, increased urine production, and increased gastric secretions (hydrochloric acid and other stomach juice components get released into the stomach even if there is no food there to digest). Long-term intake of more than 600 milligrams per day may lead to chronic insomnia, persistent anxiety, paranoia, depression, and stomach upset. (A 5-oz cup of coffee yields from 66 to 112 mg of caffeine, depending on how it is made. A cup of tea contains over 25 mg; some sodas, about 50. See Exercise 3 of chapter 10 for a precise breakdown.)

The results of studies on whether or not caffeine is a risk factor for cardiovascular disease and some cancers have been mixed. According to some sources, it's the boiled type of coffee Europeans drink that may raise cholesterol levels; the filtered coffee we drink here in the United States is currently not being charged with this crime. We do know, however, that caffeine quickens respiration, raises blood pressure, stimulates the kidneys (it's a diuretic), stimulates the digestive system (vitamins may go through the intestines without the chance to be absorbed), and excites brain function (that's the caffeine rush).

The bottom line is that, if you're a woman over 50, there are several reasons to limit your intake of caffeine (and opt for decaffeinated beverages)—although none of them are life-threatening. Specifically, limiting your intake of caffeine may help you to:

- Be more comfortable during menopause.
- Maintain your hydration better (and avoid dehydration).
- Keep your energy more constant by avoiding highs and quick drops in your blood sugar levels.
- Minimize any loss of calcium in the urine. Caffeine has been linked to calcium excretion in the urine. Mind you, caffeine's effect on urinary calcium may be most pronounced when calcium intake is low. Nevertheless, it is yet one more reason to keep your caffeine consumption in check.

Why Limit Your Intake of Alcohol?

Let's hope it's obvious why it is best, for men and women alike, not to drink too much alcohol. But here are a few reasons why women over 50, in particular, should limit their intake of alcoholic beverages:

- Alcohol provides empty calories, and most postmenopausal women can't afford to consume too many empty calories. They need to get their calories from foods that contribute vital nutrients.
- Alcohol reduces the body's ability to absorb calcium via the intestine. It may also interfere with the bone-protecting benefits of estrogen.
- The body considers alcohol a toxic substance. It tries to metabolize or excrete it as quickly as possible (thus it's not a good source of energy). When consumed in excess of our immediate energy needs, alcohol calories are likely to be converted to fat for storage.

To some extent, how much alcohol you decide to drink is a personal matter. What's excessive for one person may be quite different for another. So far, no one has gone out on a limb to claim how much alcohol, exactly, is too much for postmenopausal women. But the U.S. Dietary Guidelines recommend that women in general drink no more than one alcoholic drink a day (5 oz of wine, $1\frac{1}{2}$ oz of hard liquor, or 12 oz of beer).

Why Do We Need to Drink Water?

Just as carbohydrates are the body's fuel of choice, water is the body's preferred beverage, especially as we grow older. There are really three reasons for this.

1. *Estrogen-deficient tissues, particularly in the urinary tract, are more susceptible to infection.* This means women have an increased risk of urinary-tract infections during and after menopause. Not only is it a good idea, therefore, to drink an occasional glass of cranberry juice, but it's also important to provide your kidneys with plenty of water and to avoid diuretics (like caffeine and alcohol) so the bladder stays active and any bacteria in the bladder or urinary tract stay well diluted.

2. Diet Commandment #9 suggests that you increase your fiber consumption to 20 to 30 grams a day. *And a crucial component of increasing your fiber intake is also increasing your fluid intake, preferably water.* This will help minimize any blockages in the intestines and will help keep things running smoothly in that department, in general.

3. *As we age, our thirst mechanism isn't what it used to be.* We may really be on the verge of mild dehydration and not feel thirsty. So, in an effort to keep our bodies well hydrated, you shouldn't wait to feel thirsty to go for that cup of water.

THE BOTTOM LINE ON DIET AND OSTEOPOROSIS

Even if you decide not to take estrogen, you can still reduce your post-menopausal bone loss by:

- Consuming 1,500 milligrams of calcium every day.
- Consuming 400 IU of vitamin D every day (but not much more than half of that from a supplement).
- Doing 45 to 60 minutes of weight-bearing exercise four times a week. (Remember, only weight-bearing exercise, not swimming or bicycling, directly benefits bone mass).
- Eating foods and food components that can help your body absorb the calcium you do consume, a group that includes not only vitamin D but also lactose, magnesium, and boron.
- Avoiding foods and food components that encourage bone and calcium loss, especially excessive animal protein, excessive caffeine, alcohol, and carbonated soft drinks.
- Discussing other approaches with your doctor if you are at high risk for osteoporosis. Some possibilities are **calcitonin injections** (a calcium-regulating hormone approved by the FDA for treating osteoporosis), etidronate, and fluoride (still considered experimental).

8

IT'S NEVER TOO LATE: PREVENTING CANCER AND HEART DISEASE

Statistics show that most of us will live well into our seventies and eighties. So you'll probably have many years left to benefit from starting to eat defensively now. Not only will you feel better right now, but you'll likely live longer and feel better during that longer life. You want to be as disease-free and feel as youthful as possible with each passing birthday. Eating right can't *guarantee* this, but it sure helps put the odds in your favor. Of course, earlier is better when it comes to eating right, but at any age you can increase your muscle mass, reverse fatty deposits in your arteries, and eat foods that are known to help prevent cancer. This chapter will tell you how.

KNOW YOUR RISKS— AND HOW YOU CAN REDUCE THEM

Growing older increases everyone's risk of heart disease and cancer, but more so for women than for men, because after menopause a woman's heart disease risk profile starts resembling that of a man's. And that's not good. The estrogen women produce before menopause helps raise their levels of HDL ("good") cholesterol and lower their levels of LDL ("bad") cholesterol in the blood. Once estrogen production declines, however, this protective factor is gone. One in nine women aged 45 to 64 have some form of cardiovascular disease. By age 65, this portion skyrockets to one in three.

Some of us are more likely to develop heart disease than others. Your risk is higher if you (1) have high blood cholesterol levels, (2) have high blood pressure, (3) smoke, (4) are diabetic, or (5) have a family history of premature heart disease (defined as heart disease before age 55). You can do something about the first three of these five risk factors. You can make dietary and lifestyle changes to help lower your cholesterol levels and high blood pressure (which may include enlisting the aid of appropriate medications in addition to dietary modifications). And if you smoke, you can stop. Moreover, there is yet another powerful predictor for heart disease that you can do something about—excess body weight. Carrying extra fat around also increases your risk of hypertension, diabetes, and increased levels of LDL (bad) cholesterol and triglycerides, all considered risk factors for heart disease. Excess body weight is also thought to increase your chance of breast cancer.

Risk factors for cancer depend, in part, on the type of cancer. But overall, your risk is higher if you smoke, drink excessive amounts of alcohol, or eat a diet that's high in fat and low in fiber, fruits, and vegetables.

You may hear or read about **"heart-healthy"** diets and **"anticancer"** diets. Relax; don't let these terms confuse you. They're really *not* two different diets. Thankfully, many dietary suggestions serve both goals. Evidence now indicates that following a few dietary suggestions can help prevent both of these two top killers. Essentially, you should:

- Eat a diet low in saturated fats.
- Avoid obesity—especially abdominal (or apple-shaped) obesity.
- Eat more folic acid, omega-3 fatty acids, and possibly eat more soy protein.

Further, you can reduce your risk of both heart disease and cancer by consuming lots of antioxidant-rich foods—namely, fruits and vegetables.

ANTIOXIDANTS HELP PROTECT YOUR BODY

Though many vitamins and minerals promote health, several vitamins play particularly strong roles in protecting your body from damage that can lead to disease. These nutrients as a group are called **antioxidants,** and they are:

- Vitamin C.
- Vitamin E.
- Beta-carotene (a chemical cousin of vitamin A).

How You Can Fight Oxidation

Researchers discovered only recently that oxygen damage to your cells seems to be partly responsible for the effects of aging and chronic disease. Since **oxidation** is harmful, it makes sense that antioxidants would be beneficial. These are the substances that protect against oxygen damage by neutralizing the harmful effects of **free radicals.**

Free radicals have been implicated in a range of fatal diseases and in the process of aging itself. In the laboratory, free radicals have been shown to disrupt and actually tear apart important cell structures like membranes and genes. As a result, the individual owning the cells is more likely to develop cancer, heart disease, cataracts, and some nerve diseases.

What makes free radicals? Free radicals are produced by normal body processes and common external hazards such as ultraviolet (UV) light, X-rays and other radiation, heat, cigarette smoke, alcohol, and some pollutants. Although there is no way to stop your body from occasionally producing free radicals, you can fight their effects in two ways.

1. *Limit your exposure to the external hazards.* Wear sunscreen, long sleeves, and hats when outside. Stop smoking, and avoid secondhand smoke. Drink alcohol in moderation, if at all.

2. *Consume foods rich in antioxidants.* Antioxidants protect us by donating electrons to stabilize and neutralize the harmful effects of free radicals. Antioxidants have the ability not only to control wayward free radicals but even to repair the molecular mayhem they often produce. Different antioxidants do different jobs: Some deactivate free radicals; others transform them to less toxic compounds.

Fortunately, antioxidants aren't hard to get. Most are found in abundance in our friends, the fruit and vegetable group.

Antioxidants As Disease Prevention Weapons

Scientists first looked at antioxidants as anticancer weapons. This approach has shown promise, though not all results are in. Now researchers are finding evidence that these same nutrients may help reduce the risk of heart disease as well.

Antioxidants and Cancer Prevention

Several studies have strongly pointed to a connection between antioxidants in foods or supplements and reduced cancer risk. These studies show that people whose blood or diets contain high levels of beta-carotene appear to have a lower risk of developing lung cancer. Those with high levels of vitamin C appear to have a lower risk of stomach cancer. And in animal studies, **canthaxanthin** (a carotenoid), in conjunction with vitamin A and several other related compounds, appears to reduce the incidence of breast tumors.

In a groundbreaking study in North-Central China, reported in the 1993 issue of *Journal of the National Cancer Institute,* participants were given either a daily supplement containing from one to two times the RDA of beta-carotene, vitamin E, and selenium, or a placebo. The subsequent cancer rate of those taking the antioxidant supplement was 13 percent lower than those in the control group.

The most versatile cancer-fighting antioxidant is vitamin C. After examining over 90 epidemiological studies, a renowned researcher, Gladys Block, reported in the *American Journal of Clinical Nutrition* that she found "strong evidence" for vitamin C having protective effects on the esophagus, oral cavity, stomach, and pancreas, and "somewhat strong" evidence for it protecting against cervical, breast, and rectal cancers.

Despite these results, there have also been studies that show no relation between antioxidants and cancer prevention, particularly when supplements are used. One of the more recent such studies tested 850 people divided into four different groups with supplements of (1) beta-carotene, (2) vitamins C and E, (3) all three antioxidants, or (4) a placebo. The people in the study were mostly men with one previous colon **polyp** (a benign intestinal growth that can be a forerunner to colon cancer). No differences were seen among the groups in the number of new polyps found over the next 4 years. While this study doesn't necessarily prove that there is no link between antioxidants and colon cancer, it certainly suggests that these three antioxidants alone are not the answer to all our disease woes. There may be additional beneficial substances, such as **flavonoids,** which are also found in fruits and vegetables, that weren't given to the study participants.

Antioxidants and Heart Disease Prevention

The possible connection between antioxidants and lower cancer risk is not new information. But a Harvard researcher, Joann Manson, M.D., recently found preliminary evidence that women who eat a relatively large amount of antioxidant-rich foods also have a lower risk of heart attack (a 33 percent lower risk) and stroke (a 71 percent lower risk) than other women. Indeed, the evidence supporting the benefits of eating more fruits and vegetables is quite solid.

Boston researchers recently studied the diets of 8,700 female nurses and discovered that it's not an apple but a carrot a day that really keeps the doctor away. They found that the nurses who ate five or more servings of carrots a week were 68 percent less likely to suffer a stroke than those who ate no more than one serving a month. Carrots, of course, are one of the richest food sources of beta-carotene.

A recent USDA study reported in the *American Journal of Clinical Nutrition* shed even more light on the link between antioxidants and heart disease. Women over 58 who consumed 120 to 180 milligrams of vitamin C (that is, two to three times the RDA) had almost three times the blood levels of HDL (good) cholesterol than people who consumed less. But the blood concentrations of vitamin C weren't any higher for those women consuming more than 215 milligrams a day. This finding may indicate that 215 milligrams is the daily threshold for vitamin C consumption.

Scientists theorize that antioxidants help prevent heart disease because LDL (bad) cholesterol damages the lining of the arteries when it becomes oxidized. However, antioxidants may help protect against this oxidation by neutralizing free radicals. The truth is that although much of the findings sound promising, researchers are still in the process of understanding which antioxidants help protect us from which diseases, how the processes work, and what combinations and amounts are effective. Results from ongoing clinical trials will be coming in as early as 1996, perhaps giving us more insight into the role of antioxidant supplements and antioxidant-rich foods in the treatment and prevention of heart disease.

The Bottom Line on Antioxidants: Food before Supplements

One study concludes that we should "take antioxidant supplements." Two weeks later, another study reports that "antioxidant supplements don't help—they may even hurt." What's a health-conscious person to do? Perhaps you are in the wrong aisle of your supermarket. Instead of relying on vitamin-mineral supplements to ward off chronic diseases, go to the produce department and stock up on fruits and vegetables. Until further notice, this is still the best place to get your antioxidants. And instead of gambling on which antioxidant you are going to place your bets on, and in what amounts, try some old-fashioned sources of at least two antioxidants (vitamin C and beta-carotene), already balanced and in the nature-made combinations of fruits and vegetables. (Of course, some fruits and vegetables are higher in certain antioxidants than others. For specific information, see Tables 9.4 and 10.2.)

Chances are, other protective substances in foods complement the protective effects of antioxidants (or perhaps act independently). Thus, when we get our antioxidants from antioxidant-rich foods (rather than from vitamin-mineral supplements), we are most likely consuming these other possible protective substances as well. For example, flavonoids are a huge class of antioxidantlike substances also commonly found in fruits and vegetables. Dutch researchers recently discovered that the people who ate the most flavonoids in their diet had a 68 percent lower risk of dying from heart disease than those who ate the least (after accounting for other known risk factors). Flavonoids might act by reducing the formation of oxidized LDL (bad) cholesterol and thus reducing the growth of fatty deposits (plaque) in the arteries. The major food sources of flavonoids in the Dutch diet are onions and apples.

Although most experts agree that *foods* rich in antioxidants may indeed offer protection against some forms of cancer, heart disease, and strokes, as well as slow the aging process, National Cancer Institute researchers say it's too early to make a public health recommendation to take antioxidant *sup-*

plements. Experts at the Food and Drug Administration (FDA) are saying essentially the same thing—and in addition believe that health claims for antioxidant supplements are not yet warranted. This brings us to another Diet Commandment.

DIET COMMANDMENT #7

Eat Several Antioxidant-Rich Foods Every Day

Vitamin E, the Other Antioxidant

Over the years, vitamin E has taken a backseat to the other antioxidants, beta-carotene and vitamin C, which continue to share the spotlight. Vitamin E was sometimes added to lists that named all the antioxidants, almost as an afterthought, although in the early 1980s vitamin E supplementation was mentioned as a possible therapy for fibrocystic breast disease. But, as it turns out, vitamin E has its own identity and health benefits, apart from the other, better-known antioxidants.

What Vitamin E Can Do for You That the Other Antioxidants Can't
Regarding heart disease prevention, a report done by the University of Texas and the Dallas Medical Center concluded that, "Vitamin E appears to be the most potent antioxidant for LDL, bad cholesterol, oxidation." This is very exciting information since LDL oxidation is associated with diseases of the arteries.

Regarding cancer prevention, vitamin E is thought to work like the other antioxidants, by destroying oxygen-containing compounds, which can cause cancer if not kept in check. But there may also be something extra vitamin E can do to help protect us from cancer. Although research on this is not yet definitive, it also appears, from animal studies only, that a synthetic form of vitamin E (**vitamin E succinate**) may act like a hormone by sending a message to cancer cells to stop their growth. Apparently, vitamin E succinate actually interrupts the cancer cell's ability to divide and reproduce. Even small doses of this synthetic form quickly boosted the production of white blood cells (strengthening immunity). And in laboratory tests, vitamin E succinate was successful in fighting a wide variety of tumor cells.

Getting Your Vitamin E
In terms of reducing heart disease risk, recent studies suggest that it takes at least 100 IU (67 mg) of vitamin E per day to see results. The problem is, you can't get that much vitamin E from food, especially not on a low-fat diet. The best food sources of vitamin E are vegetable oils used in cooking. Table 8.1

Table 8.1. Vegetable Oils Richest and Poorest in Vitamin E

Vegetable Oil	Vitamin E Content (IU/Tbsp)
Richest	
Barley oil	20.4
Corn oil	14.0 (or less)*
Soybean oil	14.0 (or less)*
Canola (rapeseed) oil	8.9 (or less)*
Cottonseed oil	8.9 (or less)*
Sunflower oil	8.6
Safflower oil	6.4
Poorest	
Sesame oil	3.9
Peanut oil	3.4 (or less)*
Olive oil	1.8

*For these oils, ranges of vitamin E content are available from vitamin E researchers, not precise amounts. For the purposes of this table, I've listed the high end of the range of possible vitamin E content. So the actual vitamin E content may be slightly less, depending on the particular source or brand of the oil.

lists which vegetable oils are richest and poorest in vitamin E. For other plant sources of vitamin E, see Table 9.4.

All in all, for the best antioxidant protection, you might need to take a vitamin E supplement. But how much? We don't yet know the optimal amount for preventing disease, but the level of vitamin E supplementation suggested to avoid premenstrual syndrome (PMS) symptoms is 300 to 400 IU per day. However, this guideline is based on only a few studies (and primarily anecdotal evidence), which showed significant improvement in a variety of PMS symptoms with no side effects.

Some experts, observing the effects of vitamin E on immune function, have set the vitamin E supplementation level a little higher: 400 to 800 IU a day. In one recent study, reported in *Nutrition Reviews,* adults who took 800 IU of vitamin E for a month showed improvements in several immune function measurements. And in two large clinical trials going on right now, two levels of vitamin E supplementation are being tested, 400 IU and 600 IU. What should you do until the results of these studies become available? Taking 400 IU of vitamin E a day is probably an effective and safe choice. There are no known dangers of vitamin E supplementation at this level.

OTHER PLANT-BASED DISEASE FIGHTERS

Plant-based foods give us antioxidants and the most beneficial cooking oils, but plant-based foods can do even more to help reduce your risk of cancer and heart disease. We'll now discuss some of the beneficial effects of folic acid and phytochemicals.

Folic Acid: The B Vitamin That Thinks It's an Antioxidant

Folic acid may just be the most promising of the B vitamins when it comes to preventing disease. Folic acid hit the front page of newspapers in the early 1990s when controlled trials confirmed that when pregnant women took in more folic acid during the crucial first 6 weeks of pregnancy, their newborns had a three- to fourfold reduction in neural tube defects.

Folic Acid and Cancer Protection

Now folic acid is being credited as a possible protector against cancer. According to Harvard Medical School researchers, folic acid may be one of the key ingredients in fruits and vegetables that helps prevent colon cancer, possibly by assisting in the process that turns cancer genes off. Take note, however, that alcohol intake, the Harvard researchers added, appears to block folic acid's action and may *promote* cancer. Other studies also show that poor folic acid intake and moderate to excessive alcohol consumption have been associated with increased risk of colorectal cancer.

There is a thin line between substances that help protect the body from cancer—perhaps through blocking actions or other processes not yet determined—and substances that help strengthen the immune system. After all, one of the primary functions of the body's immune system is to react to cells or substances that are foreign, or potentially damaging, to the body. Cancer cells are among these. The healthy immune system uses several strategies to destroy cancer cells.

In addition to its specific cancer-fighting functions, folic acid has been shown to enhance many aspects of immunity. In addition, a deficiency of folic acid appears to weaken the body's immunity, its antibody responses, and its resistance to infections. Results in this field are still considered controversial, but certainly eating the recommended daily amount of folic acid from fruits and vegetables is a good way to help keep your immune system strong.

How Folic Acid and Vitamin B-6 May Protect Your Heart

Along with folic acid, vitamin B-6's role in preventing heart disease is just beginning to be understood. A recent study showed an association between low dietary intakes and blood levels of these vitamins with high blood levels of a chemical linked to clogged arteries (**homocysteine**). The people in the study who had the highest intakes of folic acid and vitamin B-6 (two times the RDA), had the lowest blood levels of this chemical. In another recent study, it took at least two times the RDA of folic acid and 1.3 times the RDA of vitamin B-6 to significantly lower the dangerous levels of homocysteine.

Getting Your Folic Acid

National food consumption surveys reveal that half the nation's women do not eat adequate amounts of folic acid in their daily diets. The amount of folic acid recommended daily (as revised in 1989) is 180 micrograms for women over the age of 15. Folic acid is found primarily in leafy green vegetables, legumes, some fruits, and, to a lesser extent, whole grains. (A good way to remember this is to think "foliage" when you think of folic acid.) Vitamin B-6 is found in fruits and vegetables and whole grains, as well as chicken, fish, and lean pork. The amount of vitamin B-6 recommended daily is 1.6 milligrams for women over the age of 18. If you eat at least five servings of fruits and vegetables every day, you would most likely be getting enough folic acid and vitamin B-6.

Phytochemicals: Produce Heroes

An important new area in nutrition research concerns **phytochemicals.** By definition, phytochemicals are chemicals found in plants. (Recall that *phyto* comes from a Greek word meaning "plant.") The study of plant chemicals is quite promising because these nature-made substances can be very powerful in terms of cancer prevention and other important health benefits.

How Phytochemicals Protect You

Thousands of these chemicals evolved in plants to protect them from the ravages of sunlight, and they can benefit you, too. Scientists have found that phytochemicals somehow disable the processes involved in cancerous cell growth. The cancer never gets a chance to start. Each phytochemical helps protect the body from cancer in its own way: Some escort carcinogens out of body cells; others trigger enzymes that combat carcinogens. Some keep carcinogens from damaging DNA; others keep cancer cells from multiplying. Although we still have much to learn about phytochemicals, the preliminary discoveries are very exciting.

One phytochemical, **indole-3-carbinol** (found in broccoli and other cruciferous vegetables such as bok choy, Brussels sprouts, cabbage, cauliflower, Chinese cabbage, greens, kale, kohlrabi, rutabagas, and turnips), has already been proven to inhibit tumor growth in laboratory animals. Indole-3-carbinol is only one of many known phytochemicals; countless others will no doubt be discovered. However, if you eat the foods containing the phytochemicals that we *do* know about, you will probably also consume some of the phytochemicals we don't yet know about. This is yet another reason to get our nutrition in the balanced and complete forms found in natural foods—fruits, vegetables, and beans—not from pills or powders.

Getting Your Phytochemicals

Phytochemicals can be found in an assortment of plant foods. Beans and bean products, for example, contain four known phytochemicals: **protease inhibitors**, which suppress enzyme production in cancer cells to slow tumor growth; **phytosterols**, which hinder cell reproduction in the large intestine, possibly preventing colon cancer; **isoflavones,** which block estrogen from entering cells, possibly reducing the risk of breast and ovarian cancer; and **saponins**, which interfere with DNA replication, preventing cancer cells from multiplying. Grains contain **phytic acid,** which binds to iron, possibly preventing the creation of cancer-causing free radicals. But probably the largest plant sources of phytochemicals are fruits and vegetables.

In addition to being found in an assortment of plant foods, phytochemicals can be arranged or classified into four general types, according to their functions or effects: (1) those that act as antioxidants, (2) those that mimic the effects of estrogen (known as **phytoestrogens;** see chapter 3), (3) those that act as blocking agents, and (4) those that act as enzyme inducers. Table 9.1 (in the next chapter) lists fruits and vegetables rich in phytoestrogens (and also boron); Table 9.4 lists a wide variety of foods rich in antioxidants; and Table 8.2 (here) lists several of the recently discovered phytochemicals that fall into the latter two categories, serving as blocking agents and enzyme inducers (though some also have antioxidant properties), along with their known fruit and vegetable sources. The demonstrated effects listed in this table are based only on animal and test-tube studies—not on studies with people. But even if the research is only preliminary, we know you can't go wrong by eating the fruits and vegetables mentioned in this table—especially those that get mentioned repeatedly.

FATS AND DISEASE PREVENTION

Watching your intake of fats with an eye toward preventing cancer and heart disease can be both complicated and simple. Complicated, because lots of components in fats can adversely affect your health, including cholesterol, *trans* fatty acids, and saturated fats. But simple, because eating a low-fat diet provides protection from all of these.

The Rights and Wrongs of Cholesterol

Your body contains two kinds of cholesterol: the easily oxidized low-density lipoproteins, known as LDL, or "bad" cholesterol, and high-density lipopro-

Table 8.2. Some Recently Discovered Phytochemicals, Their Demonstrated Effects, and Their Sources

Phytochemical (or Group)	Demonstrated Effects	Vegetable Sources	Fruit Sources
Sulphoraphane and other isothiocyanates	Stimulate production of anticancer enzymes, boosting the body's cancer-fighting abilities.	Broccoli, Brussels sprouts, cabbage, cauliflower, kale, kohlrabi, and turnips	
Phenolic acids (ellagic, p-coumaric, and chlorogenic acid)	Inhibit formation of nitrosamine (a carcinogen) and affect enzyme activity. Also have some antioxidant properties.	Carrots, peppers, and tomatoes	Apples, grapes, pineapple, raspberries, and strawberries
Allyl sulfides	Block the action of carcinogenic chemicals. (Other allium compounds may decrease the production of tumor cells.)	Chives, garlic, leeks, and onions	
Terpenes (monoterpene and limonene)	Step up production of enzymes that may help dispose of potent carcinogens. Also have some antioxidant properties.	Broccoli, cabbage, carrots, cucumbers, eggplant, garlic, peppers, squash, tomatoes, and yams	Apples and citrus fruits
3-N-butyl phthalide	Active in tumor inhibition.	Celery and parsley (the only confirmed sources)	
Capsaicin	Keeps carcinogens from binding to DNA, where they can trigger changes that lead to lung and other cancers.	Chili peppers	

	Function	Vegetable sources	Fruit sources
Carotenoids (This group includes lutein, which is green; beta-carotene, which is orange; and lycopene, which is red.)	Function as antioxidants and cell-differentiation agents (cancer cells are nondifferentiated). (lycopene has been associated with decreased incidences of pancreatic and cervical cancers.)	Carrots, kale, spinach, sweet potatoes, tomatoes, greens in general, winter squash, and yams	Apricots, cantaloupe, watermelon, and citrus fruits
Catechins (tannins)	Function as antioxidants somehow (exact mechanism not yet known, but linked to lower rates of intestinal cancer.)	Green tea	Bananas, berries, and strawberries
Plant sterols	Function as cell-differentiation agents (cancer cells are nondifferentiated).	Broccoli, cabbage, cucumbers, eggplant, peppers, squash, tomatoes, and yams	Bananas and cantaloupe

teins, known as HDL, or "good" cholesterol. Before menopause, women naturally tend to have higher levels of HDL, but after menopause the HDL level normally drops. In fact, it takes only 6 to 10 years (after the onset of menopause) for a woman's risk of heart disease to catch up to a man's—which tells us that after menopause, it's even *more* important to work at raising our HDL levels.

How do you increase your HDL levels while lowering your LDL levels? The best methods are as follows:

- Get regular aerobic exercise.
- Eat a low-fat diet.
- Include monounsaturated fats and omega-3 fatty acids as part of your low-fat diet.
- Avoid *trans* fatty acids.
- Maintain a healthy weight.

Some of that advice is clear and familiar; some may seem, at first glance, to be rather complicated. How many different types of fats are there? Bear with me, and we'll sort it all out.

The Saturation Confusion

Saturated, partially saturated (or hydrogenated), polyunsaturated, monounsaturated, *trans* fatty acids—these are all terms we not only hear about in the news but also see on many food packages. But what do they all mean?

Saturated Fat

This kind of fatty acid holds as many hydrogen atoms as it has room for. Most animal fats, like butter and cream, are saturated fats. But many margarines become saturated, too, thanks to a process called **hydrogenation.** A few plant-based oils (palm oil, palm kernel oil, and coconut oil) are also naturally saturated.

Your consumption of saturated fats should be kept to a minimum since they are associated with heart disease when eaten in higher amounts. They may also be associated with cancer. In a recent study published in the *Journal of the National Cancer Institute,* researchers looked at diet and cancer in a new way. They looked at how women ate *before* they were diagnosed with breast cancer and what result their diet had on their cancer *survival.* The study's results suggested that women with higher intakes of saturated fat had an increased risk of dying from the breast cancer. There is also evidence that saturated fat may increase the risk of ovarian and colon cancers.

Partially Hydrogenated Fat

This is fat that has been only partially saturated with hydrogen atoms. Hydrogenation is the process of forcing hydrogen into unsaturated oils, often to make them more solid and to prolong their shelf life. These fats are partially saturated, so they too should be eaten in moderation.

Polyunsaturated Fat

These fats are usually liquid at room temperature. Examples are cottonseed, saffola, soy, and corn oils. Since too much fat in the diet, overall, can encourage disease, even polyunsaturated fats should not be used liberally.

Monounsaturated Fat

These fats are usually liquid at room temperature. Examples are canola and olive oil. Of all the fats, this type has been shown to offer the most health benefits. Monounsaturated fats seem to provide good protection from heart disease. Replacing saturated fats with mostly monounsaturated fats (for example, using olive or canola oil in cooking instead of butter, margarine, or shortening) apparently minimizes the unwanted decrease in the good cholesterol (HDL) that often occurs when you lower the total amount of fat in your diet.

Trans *Fatty Acids*

When vegetable oils are partially hydrogenated, some of the molecules convert into a new configuration, (a *trans* configuration—hence the name). These ***trans* fatty acids** have been shown to raise blood levels of LDL (bad) cholesterol while also lowering blood levels of HDL (good) cholesterol—neither of which is a desirable goal.

At the heart of the *trans* fatty acid issue is the debate over which is better, as part of a low-fat diet, butter or margarine. Both stick margarine and butter have about the same grams of fat per tablespoon. Most margarine contains its share of saturated fats, some of which are *trans* fatty acids. Butter also contains saturated fat but adds some cholesterol into the equation. Butter is probably fine if used in moderation; people tend to use a lot more margarine to compensate for its weaker (than butter) taste. It's probably better, though, to use a little butter than a lot of margarine.

Trans fatty acids also occur in partially hydrogenated vegetable oils and in many processed foods that are high in *trans* fats, such as chips, puddings, crackers, cookies, and other high-fat baked goods. Buy the lower-fat options in these product categories, and you automatically lower the amount of *trans* fats you'll be eating.

Omega-3s Fatty Acids

Even within each of the different categories of fats, there are many different types of fats. Within the polyunsaturated group, for instance, a particular type of fat has been identified as playing a special protective role in the body, the **omega-3 fatty acids.** Omega-3s have been linked to lowering both blood pressure and serum triglyceride levels (triglycerides account for 90 percent of the fat we get from food), preventing blood clots (thereby decreasing the chance of stroke) and the closing of blood vessels following vascular surgery. They may even help increase HDL (good) cholesterol levels. But omega-3s don't just fight heart disease. They have also been shown to slow or prevent cancerous tumor growth as well as reducing symptoms of inflammatory diseases such as rheumatoid arthritis. The two particular cancers that omega-3s may help prevent are colon and possibly breast cancer.

All of this means that when you do use fat, it's a good idea to use an omega-3 source when possible. The two most important omega-3 fatty acids are **EPA (eicosapentaenoic acid)** and **DHA (docosahexaenoic acid).** Fatty fish such as sardines, herring, anchovies, whitefish and bluefish, salmon, and mackerel are the best known food sources of omega-3 fatty acids. Swordfish, canned tuna, rainbow trout, striped bass, pacific oysters, and squid are fair sources.

But eating lots of fish isn't the easiest habit to get into for many of us, especially if you live in the midwest or don't have a seafood shop or restaurant that you trust nearby. Have no fear, though: Vegetables, soybeans, and seeds are here. Some plant foods contain **alpha-linolenic acid,** which the body can partially convert to the omega-3 fatty acid known as EPA. You will find alpha-linolenic acid in linseed oil, walnuts and walnut oil, flaxseed, rapeseed (used to make canola oil), soybeans, spinach, and mustard greens.

Some words of caution: Eating too much fish (on a daily basis) can depress immune function. Overdosing on fatty fish or fish oil can also be harmful if you have bleeding problems because it can interfere with anticoagulant medicines. Further, high doses of fish oil (mainly from fish oil pills) may increase insulin requirements in diabetics.

Now we get to omega-3's alter ego, the **omega-6 fatty acids.** Omega-6 fatty acids are found in vegetable oils like corn, safflower, and sunflower oil. Omega-6 fatty acids compete with the omega-3s for control of many biochemical reactions in the body. When omega-6s are in a much higher proportion than omega-3s, an overproduction of hormonelike substances (**prostaglandins** and **leukotrienes**) can result, which can encourage plaque buildup on artery walls, disrupt the immune system, and form blood clots.

Because of this ongoing battle between the omega fatty acids, some researchers suggest we eat about equal amounts of omega-3s and omega-6s. In contrast, the typical American diet has a dangerous 10 to 1 ratio of omega-6s to omega-3s. Here are four things you can do to quickly improve your omega fatty acid ratio:

1. Eat fish two or three times a week.
2. Switch to canola oil or soybean oil for cooking; switch to brands of nonstick sprays that use one of these two oils.
3. Limit your use of salad dressings, margarine, mayonnaise, and vegetable oils unless they are high in omega-3 fatty acids.
4. Eat more soybeans and soybean products, spinach, and mustard greens.

A Low-Fat Diet Is the Key

Switching to canola oil is certainly one step in the right direction, but the best way to alter your fat consumption to prevent disease is to eat less fat overall. Let us not forget that any fat, in excess, is a bad fat—even olive oil and canola oil. It's all too easy to simply switch our fat, from butter to margarine, or from shortening to vegetable oil. Television commercials are telling you it's all right to eat fat and fry chicken—as long as you use their oil. Fast-food chains are telling you that their french fries are fried in all-vegetable oil, so eat up! But don't forget, vegetable oil is 100 percent fat. Each tablespoon contains 13.5 grams of fat.

When you eat a low-fat diet, you will likely keep your intake of saturated fat, *trans* fatty acids, and omega-6 fatty acids low as well. But a low-fat diet may inadvertently lower the HDL (good) cholesterol level in your blood while it's also lowering the LDL (bad) cholesterol level. Fortunately, monounsaturated fats (canola and olive oils) as your primary fat source seem to keep HDL levels from dropping.

In summary, (1) use less fat overall; (2) when you do use fat, use an omega-3 source that is also a monounsaturated fat, like canola oil; and (3) use olive oil, a monounsaturated fat, when a highly flavored oil is needed. And how do we quantify "less fat overall"? The answer is important enough to be the next Diet Commandment.

DIET COMMANDMENT #8

Eat No More Than 20 to 25 Percent of Your Calories from Fat

When a blood vessel is so narrow from fatty deposits that a blood clot forms, completely blocking the flow of blood to the heart, a heart attack results. When the blood vessels to your brain are clogged, you can suffer a stroke. Either one is serious trouble. Recent advances in our understanding of clot formation and blood protein factors may identify (or help identify) the missing risk factors for heart disease. All these answers point directly to the importance of a low-fat diet. According to very recent research (although done on men, it should apply to menopausal women as well), hours after we eat a fat-rich meal, we are at a higher risk of fatal heart attacks than at other times, because fatty meals appear to increase levels of a protein factor involved with clotting (**thrombosis**). In one study, men who got 50 percent of their calories from fat had higher levels of this clotting factor than men who got only 20 percent of their calories from fat. In another study of men who have already had heart bypass surgery, researchers found that further damage to the heart arteries could be reduced, and that in some cases partially blocked blood vessels could even begin to open, when the men took drugs to lower their cholesterol levels and ate a low-fat diet.

What's a Butter Lover to Do?

Because eating a low-fat diet is the ultimate answer, an indiscriminate use of butter or margarine is still a nutritional no-no. Ask yourself whether you would use less fat at the table if that fat was butter; or would you still glob it on? If you are a relentless globber, perhaps you are better off with one of the diet margarines, although preferably one with an ingredient label that reads, "water, liquid canola oil," rather than "partially hydrogenated canola oil." However, if you can spread butter like it's gold (or something equally precious), you may be better off with butter.

Much Ado about the Mediterranean Diet

The typical Mediterranean diet is vastly different from the typical American diet. Think of authentic Greek and Italian cuisines. People following such a diet eat more bread, more root and green vegetables, more fish, and more fruit. They also eat less red meat (poultry is often eaten in place of beef, lamb, and pork) and less butter and cream (rapeseed or canola oil and olive oils are used more often).

A few research projects have tried putting non-Mediterranean people on a simulated typical Mediterranean diet. In one such study, the experimental group ate more alpha-linolenic acids (which can convert to heart-friendly omega-3s) and significantly less fat, saturated fat, and cholesterol than the control group. Like the typical Mediterranean diet, the experimental group's diet was rich in vegetables and fruits, supplying a nice array of antioxidants.

After a little over 2 years, there were 16 cardiac deaths in the group that didn't change to this diet compared to only three cardiac deaths and nonfatal heart attacks in the experimental group. But probably the most remarkable observation was *how quickly* the researchers could see the beneficial effects of the Mediterranean diet. After only 8 weeks, the researchers noted a reduction in recurring heart attacks, other cardiac events, and overall mortality. Moreover, this timeline confirms the 6-week period noted in a similar study. Talk about instant gratification: When it comes to heart disease prevention, it doesn't get much better than this.

A Low-Fat Diet for Cancer Prevention

The association between a high-fat diet and breast cancer is still considered controversial. But there is enough evidence and scientific theory to warrant action now. A researcher from Georgetown University, in Washington, DC, described one of the many possible connections between fat and cancer. Fat and cholesterol may be converted to estrogen precursors, which tumors may then convert to estrogen, further feeding estrogen-dependent cancers. So by eating less fat, we can significantly reduce the concentration of estrogen precursors.

Another possible connection between fat in the diet and cancer is obesity. A high-fat diet encourages the body to make and store body fat. And excessive body fat stores (that is, obesity) may increase breast cancer risk, especially after menopause. Some researchers suggest that fat intake must be less than 25 percent of calories consumed to decrease breast cancer rates. A low-fat diet also seems to reduce the risk of colon cancer and perhaps ovarian cancer.

How Much Fat Can I Have?

The recommendation to eat no more than 20 to 25 percent of your calories from fat is a realistic one in that it takes into account people's enjoyment of foods. A stricter limit, such as no more than 10 percent of your calories from fat, is too difficult for the average person to stick with over the long haul. You can't succeed without eliminating entire food categories, like dairy and meats, as well as some staples like reduced-fat cheese or lower-fat turkey hot dogs. And frankly, it's no fun unless you have a highly skilled gourmet chef with a limitless food budget working in your kitchen.

At the same time, however, a looser recommendation for fat intake—such as the government's current guideline for the general population, which is to eat no more than 30 percent of your calories from fat—is too high if you want to lose weight, and possibly too high for optimal heart disease and cancer prevention benefits as well. Thus, the recommendation to eat no more than 20 to 25 percent of your calories from fat seeks to strike a balance between enjoyment of foods on the one hand (thereby increasing the likelihood that the recommendation will be followed consistently) and maximum health benefits on the other. Of course, if you can eat even less fat than that and still enjoy your meals, more power to you. For the rest of us, chapter 9 will offer a good deal of specific information and advice on how to achieve this goal.

FIBER AND HEART DISEASE AND CANCER

Fiber, by definition, cannot be broken down and absorbed by the human body and therefore does not contribute any calories. Why then is fiber so important? Two basic types of fiber perform two critical functions: Soluble fiber—found in oats, apples, beans, and other foods—helps reduce serum cholesterol levels. And insoluble fiber—found in wheat, vegetables, and other foods—is linked to a lowered risk of colon cancer.

Since fiber cannot be digested and absorbed into the bloodstream, it remains in the intestinal tract and becomes a component of your stool. In terms of helping prevent heart disease, the soluble fiber is thought to hold onto **bile acids** (digestive substances that help break down food fats, of which cholesterol is a component) and carry them out of the body. In terms of preventing colon cancer, experts believe that fiber helps by (1) reducing the time food waste spends in the intestinal tract before it exits for good, which reduces the amount of time potential carcinogens are in contact with the intestinal wall, and (2) diluting the bile acids, some of which may promote colon cancer.

In a recent Harvard study, the people who ate low amounts of fiber and high amounts of saturated fat were nearly four times more likely to develop colorectal **adenomas** (lesions that can lead to cancer). This is some of the first evidence we've had directly linking diet to very early stages of cancer. Furthermore, some research has suggested that **phytic acid,** a component in cereals, nuts, and seeds, could be a protective element in high-fiber foods, along with the fiber itself. Phytic acid may discourage oxidation damage to the intestinal wall and neighboring cells. All of this research leads us to the next Diet Commandment.

DIET COMMANDMENT #9

Eat 20 to 30 Grams of Fiber Every Day, from a Variety of Different Foods

---

Added Benefits of Fiber

Fiber attracts water to the digestive tract, creating stools that are softer and preventing constipation. Fiber also exercises the intestinal-tract muscles, keeping them fit and toned. These are the better-known benefits of fiber. When fiber is part of a balanced meal, it also helps modulate blood sugar levels after that meal. One researcher, working with diabetes patients, was able to lower their insulin levels by 40 to 98 percent just by making sure they ate more fiber.

Eating more fiber with breakfast can have an added bonus: helping you to eat less for lunch. When study participants ate a breakfast cereal with 11

grams of fiber per serving, they tended to eat 150 fewer calories from breakfast and lunch combined than the people who ate a breakfast cereal with no
detectable fiber. Fiber may help you feel fuller by slowing your stomach
from emptying its contents into the small intestines. When the fiber reaches
the large intestine, it can ferment and produce some bloating (also giving you
a feeling of fullness). The fiber in whole-grain cereals appears to produce
more gas. And it's even possible that the fatty acids that result from fiber fer-
mentation in the colon may help decrease your appetite. Another study noted
similar weight-control attributes, this one from eating high-fiber bread.
Those who ate high-fiber bread lost considerably more weight than those
who did not.

OTHER PIECES OF THE PUZZLE CONCERNING DIET, HEART DISEASE, AND CANCER

If you're going to pay attention to just a few dietary factors that affect disease prevention, eating a low-fat diet, rich in fiber, fruits, and vegetables, is
the way to go. However, our bodies are complex systems that suffer heart
disease and cancer in many forms. And other food-related factors have also
been identified as potential risk factors for heart disease and cancer.

Diet and Hypertension

Hypertension, or high blood pressure, is one of three major risk factors for
cardiovascular disease that are influenced in part by diet (the other two are
obesity and high blood cholesterol). Chronic high blood pressure, affecting
about a third of the American adult population, usually accompanies cardiovascular disease. The higher the blood pressure is above normal, the greater
the risk of heart disease. The normal resting blood pressure for adults aver-
ages about 120/70 mm Hg. You have high blood pressure if your blood pressure is 140/90 mm Hg or higher in at least two tests.

As postmenopausal women age, their chance of having high blood pressure surpasses that of men—even among women who had normal blood
pressure most of their lives. When you have high blood pressure, your tiny
blood vessels (**arterioles**) are constricting and blood can't easily flow
through them. Your heart has to pump harder to push the same amount of
blood through. Over time, this extra work will weaken your heart. If un-
treated, high blood pressure can damage other vital organs like your brain,
eyes, and kidneys. You are also at increased risk of having a stroke, heart attack, or congestive heart failure.

You generally don't feel symptoms when you have high blood pressure;
that's why it's often called the "silent killer." You must, therefore, get your

blood pressure checked frequently—at least every 2 years if your pressure has been normal, more frequently if it has been high. If you are diagnosed with high blood pressure, your doctor may prescribe medication to lower it. But you can also take these very effective steps to help control high blood pressure—or even prevent it in the first place.

• *Lose weight.* As your weight goes up, your blood pressure often goes up too. If your weight goes down, your blood pressure often goes down. The best and safest way to lose extra weight is to eat a low-fat diet and exercise regularly.

• *Exercise regularly.* Not only will exercise automatically help you with losing weight, but it will also improve your overall cardiovascular fitness.

• *Limit your consumption of salt and other sources of sodium.* See the next section for a thorough discussion of sodium and its effects on blood pressure.

Sodium and High Blood Pressure

This is another one of those cases where a little is necessary but too much can be harmful. Your body needs a certain amount of sodium in the blood and body tissues because sodium is an electrolyte and helps maintain fluid balance, and because it assists in both nerve transmission and muscle contraction. However, some people (although not all) develop high blood pressure when they take in too much salt. These people are called **sodium-sensitive.** People at risk might be genetically prone to sodium sensitivity, have chronic kidney disease, have one or two hypertensive parents, are Black, and are over 50. Being overweight, consuming excessive alcohol, and being physically inactive may also contribute to sodium sensitivity.

In sodium-sensitive people, clearance systems that normally dispose of extra sodium don't work as effectively. The extra sodium causes the body to release more water into the bloodstream (to help balance out the high concentration of sodium), which increases the volume of blood circulating. The higher the blood volume, the higher the blood pressure tends to be.

Salt (sodium chloride, NaCl) contains sodium. And in the typical American diet, about 95 percent of the sodium we consume comes from salt. If you just buy lower-salt products and use less salt in cooking and on the table, you would make great strides in lowering your sodium intake. The National Research Council recommendation for the maximum daily consumption of sodium is 2,400 milligrams. However, the typical daily intake in the United States is around 4,000 milligrams.

Limiting sodium and salt consumption seems to help prevent high blood pressure in sodium-sensitive people but isn't as effective in about half the hypertensive people who try it. As of now, we can only identify tendencies for sodium sensitivity; but not all people with sodium problems will fit this profile. Consequently, the entire population should moderate their sodium intake, since less sodium will do most of us no harm and possibly some good.

The Case against Sugar

The same can be said about sugar: Eating less will do us no harm and possibly some good. A sizable portion of the population, especially as we age, seems to have difficultly managing high levels of sugar in the blood, meaning that the threat of diabetes must be taken seriously. At the same time, people over 50 (especially women) need more nutrients but fewer calories. Thus, sugar in the diet is more than just empty calories; it's a drag on our health as well. Excess sugar is also very likely to mean excess total calories, and is therefore turned to body fat. And as we have seen, the heart does not need either extra weight or extra fat.

Such considerations lead us to the tenth and final Diet Commandment.

DIET COMMANDMENT #10

Moderate Your Intake of Sodium and Sugar

Other Minerals That Help Fight Hypertension

A number of studies suggest that other minerals, such as potassium, calcium, and magnesium, may lessen the blood pressure response to sodium in the diet. (You'll recall from chapter 7 that two of these minerals, calcium and magnesium, are significant for osteoporosis prevention as well.) Thus, avoiding hypertension is yet another reason to make sure you're getting the RDA of calcium (1,000 to 1,500 mg a day for healthy adults) and plenty of fruits and vegetables (which are good sources of potassium and magnesium).

Food Watch on Specific Cancers

Often when we think of cancer, we feel powerless against it—as though it were a deadly sickness that we just "get," depending on our luck in life. The fact is, however, that there are definite things you can do to greatly improve your luck and reduce your risk of getting cancer. For example, the National Cancer Institute estimates that one-third of all cancer deaths may be related to the foods we eat. Specifically, the FDA believes sufficient scientific evidence exists to approve three different health claims, linking cancer prevention to a diet that is:

1. Low in fat.
2. High in fiber from grains, fruits, and vegetables.
3. Rich in fruits and vegetables, in and of themselves (in addition to the beneficial effects of fiber).

Of all of these, the diet recommendation supported by the strongest scientific evidence is to eat more fruits and vegetables.

Fruits and Vegetables and Many Types of Cancer

You just can't beat the health benefits of fruits and vegetables. Studies consistently show a decrease in cancer with an increase in fruit and vegetable consumption—in at least 15 different cancer sites. The strongest evidence shows a protective effect of fruits and vegetables on eight cancer sites: the pancreas, stomach, colon/rectum, bladder, cervix, ovary, endometrium, and breast. Indeed, Table 8.3 lists a variety of cancer-fighting dietary strategies and their demonstrated effects on cancer risks in six specific sites. These various dietary strategies are ranked in terms of how many of the six sites are affected by each one. The "Best Strategies" reduce the risk of cancer in three or more of the sites; the "Good Strategies" reduce the risk of cancer in one or two of them. It is worth noting that the only one of these dietary strategies that reduces the risk of cancer in all six sites—by far the best cancer-fighting dietary strategy you can follow—is eating more fruits and vegetables.

Looking at the relationship between fruit and vegetable consumption and cancer from the *opposite* perspective, the rate for practically every type of cancer is at least *double* among people who *don't* eat fruits and vegetables. In fact, the risk for many of these cancers might be even more than two times higher. Moreover, the evidence of the protective effects of fruits and vegetables remains strong even after considering studies conducted in 17 different countries, from China to Turkey to the United States. Many national experts speculate that there are probably several different factors in fruits and vegetables acting jointly. Bruce Ames, a well-known biochemist, believes every vitamin in food is probably part of some defense system that helps protect the body. And the only way to guarantee that you are getting each and every beneficial component of fruits and vegetables *is to eat plenty of fruits and vegetables*. (See. Your mother *was* right.)

SUMMING IT UP

The many dietary suggestions and details provided in this chapter can be summarized in a few main points, unifying the twin goals of (1) eating to help prevent heart disease and (2) eating to prevent many forms of cancer. (Several of these points also improve or benefit various other aspects of your health, both during and after menopause.) The main points to remember:

- Calcium can prevent hypertension *and* slow the onset of osteoporosis.
- A low-fat diet is vital for preventing heart disease *and* some cancers; it also discourages the accumulation of extra body fat.

Table 8.3. Dietary Strategies That Can Reduce Your Risk of Specific Cancers

Dietary Strategy	Reduces the Risk of Cancer of the					
	Breast	Lung	Ovary	Cervix	Stomach and Upper GI Tract	Colon
Best Strategies						
Eat more fruits and vegetables	✓*	✓	✓*	✓*	✓*	✓
Consume more vitamin C	✓	✓		✓	✓	
Eat less fat, especially less saturated fat	✓		✓			✓
Eat more fiber	✓		✓			✓
Consume more vitamin E	✓	✓		✓		
Consume more beta-carotene (and possibly other carotenoids)		✓		✓	✓	
Good Strategies						
Consume more vitamin A	✓	✓				
Limit your consumption of alcohol	✓					
Consume less egg cholesterol			✓			
Eat more calcium-rich foods						✓
Consume more folic acid				✓		
Consume less smoked and salted foods					✓	

*Based on the analysis of about 200 epidemiological studies (*Nutr Cancer* 18, 1–29, 1992).

- When you eat fruits and vegetables, you're definitely covering a lot of health bases: You're getting your beta-carotene, along with all the other beneficial vitamins, minerals, phytochemicals, and other protective substances yet to be discovered.
- Phytoestrogen-rich foods (phytoestrogens are one of the major types of phytochemicals) help protect your body against cancer *and* help minimize the many side effects of menopause.

The final section of this book (Part Four) shows you how to follow the 10 Diet Commandments. Chapter 9 offers tips and specific advice on how to make the 10 Diet Commandments part of your daily routine; and chapter 10 provides a method for analyzing your current eating habits against the ideal suggested by the 10 Diet Commandments.

PART FOUR

HOW TO FOLLOW THE 10 DIET COMMANDMENTS

9

MAKING THE 10 DIET COMMANDMENTS PART OF YOUR DAILY ROUTINE

This book covers a lot of territory. We've ranged from managing meno-pausal symptoms to eating for energy, then on to slowing the normal ag-ing process and helping prevent heart disease, cancer, and osteoporosis. Through it all, however, the 10 Diet Commandments reign. No matter how complicated each chapter and its information may seem, the 10 Diet Com-mandments give you a simple framework to be sure you're doing the best for your body.

The previous six chapters have presented the Diet Commandments and explained why each one is important within the context of menopausal changes. And you may have noticed that two or three different chapters often emphasize the same advice. Eating more phytoestrogen-rich foods, for ex-ample, comes up in chapters 3, 4, and 8, in the context of how to eat for a more comfortable menopause, how to up your estrogen naturally, and how to prevent heart disease and cancer.

By now you should have a good sense of why each commandment is im-portant. But how do you follow them on a daily basis? How do you make good nutritional practices part of your normal routine? This chapter provides the answers.

Instead of simply *telling* you to eat 20 to 30 grams of fiber every day, or to get at most 20 to 25 percent of your calories from fat, I'm going to *show you how* to do these things. I'm going to go through the 10 Diet Command-ments one by one, offering tables and tips to help you follow each of them. And I promise to make the process as painless, practical, and pleasureable as possible. It's true that you will probably have to change a few habits. Eating more beans and tofu, for example, may be new to you. However, I hope to ease the transition by explaining how you can incorporate canned beans and tofu into your everyday foods, and by introducing you (in appendix B) to a few recipes that are quick to fix and taste terrific.

DIET COMMANDMENT #1:
Eat at Least One Phytoestrogen-Rich Food Every Day

The two main kinds of phytoestrogens we know of so far are the isoflavonoids and the lignans. Scientists are still in the process of measuring the phytoestrogen content of various foods. So far, we know that soybeans and certain fruits and vegetables contain isoflavonoids. We can also find lignans in certain fruits and vegetables, along with certain beans, seeds, and whole grains. Thus, this commandment is basically telling us to eat more beans (especially soybeans and soybean products), fruits, and vegetables—and whole grains for lignans.

You'll find tips to help you eat more beans and tofu in the sections titled "Beans: The Wonder Food" and "Tofu Mania" later in this chapter, as well as some relevant recipes in appendix B. To learn which fruits and vegetables are rich in phytoestrogens (as well as boron), see Table 9.1. Note especially those fruits and vegetables listed in the table followed by two or even three check marks (such as broccoli and carrots): These, obviously, are especially good food choices. (For more detailed information on the phytoestrogen and boron contents of various foods, see Tables A.1, A.2, and A.3 in appendix A.)

Of course, *knowing* which fruits and vegetables are rich in phytoestrogens and actually *eating* them are two different things. Most of us already know that fruits and vegetables are good for our health and that we should be eating more of them. Actually doing it is the hard part. Diet Commandments #1 and #2 are related in that they both require, in essence, eating more fruits and vegetables. For suggestions on how to do that, see the section called "Eat 5-a-Day: It's the Sure Way" later in this chapter.

DIET COMMANDMENT #2:
Eat at Least One Boron-Rich Food Every Day

Since some amount of boron is in many common fruits and vegetables, eating at least five servings of fruits and vegetables a day will undoubtedly boost your boron totals. The fruits and vegetables particularly rich in boron are listed in Table 9.1. (For more detailed information on the boron content of various foods, see Table A.3 in appendix A.)

Note especially those fruits and vegetables listed in the table that contain both boron and one (or both) of the two major phytoestrogens: You should try to eat *two* of these fruits and vegetables each day (out of your total of five servings of fruits and vegetables daily). Or, to further simplify matters, just try to do these two things every day:

1. Eat a few stems of broccoli.
2. Eat a carrot.

When you do this, you get two foods that are rich in both phytoestrogens *and* boron. And here's a bonus: Broccoli and carrots are also rich in antioxidants and other beneficial phytochemicals.

Five Ways to Ensure a Diet Rich in Phytoestrogens and Boron

1. *Eat broccoli and carrots often.* Broccoli and carrots are extra-special vegetables in that they contain both phytoestrogens and boron. You can get your very important servings of carrots or broccoli (or both) almost every day by choosing foods or recipes that contain them, such as broccoli with pasta, low-fat cream of broccoli soup, glazed carrots, or a roast with potatoes and carrots. Or you can simply eat them straight from the refrigerator, raw and rinsed. Find the best time of day for your vegetable fix, perhaps each night as you prepare dinner. I find chewing on a raw, cold carrot or handful of broccoli cleanses my palate and helps clean my teeth before dinner. Or, if you like to make a juice concoction every day, throw a carrot into your juicer. Find the best method(s) for you, then make them a part of almost every day so that they become healthy habits.

2. *Eat a salad a day.* Many of the vegetables people normally use to make a green salad are listed in Table 9.1. Lettuce, cucumbers, bell peppers, and tomatoes are all rich in phytoestrogens and boron. So if salad appeals to you as a meal accompaniment or snack, by all means go heavy on these vegetables. But go light on the fatty salad dressing.

If fixing a salad seems like a lot of work, make a point of ordering them in restaurants or fast-food places when you go there. You can also make a big green salad just once during the week. Store it in an airtight container, and you can have fresh salad for several days. Many supermarkets now sell bags of salad fixings, washed and ready to go; all you have to do is add a few more vegetables of your own and a reduced-calorie dressing. Many supermarkets and even fast-food chains have salad bars.

You can have your salad and eat your broccoli and carrots, too. Just add sliced or grated carrots or broccoli pieces to your green salad. And here's a bonus: Eating a green salad a day may help keep hot flashes away.

3. *Get your boron from a can.* Many of the fruits containing boron (such as apricots, pears, and peaches) are available year-round—as long as you have a can opener. All three of these fruits are available canned in unsweetened juice.

Table 9.1. Common Fruits and Vegetables That Are Rich in Phytoestrogens and Boron

| | Phytoestrogens | | |
	Isoflavonoids	Lignans	Boron
Fruits			
Apples	✓		✓
Apricots			✓
Avocados			✓
Bananas			✓
Berries	✓		
Blueberries			✓
Gooseberries			✓
Red raspberries			✓
Strawberries	✓		✓
Cantaloupe			✓
Cherries, sour			✓
Citrus fruits	✓		✓
Grapefruit			✓
Oranges			✓
Figs			✓
Grapes	✓		✓
Mandarin oranges			✓
Mangoes			✓
Papaya			✓
Peaches			✓
Pears		✓	✓
Plums		✓	✓
Vegetables			
Asparagus		✓	✓
Beets		✓	✓
Bell peppers	✓	✓	✓
Broccoli	✓	✓	✓
Brussels sprouts	✓	✓	✓
Cabbage	✓	✓	✓
Carrots	✓	✓	✓

Table 9.1. (continued)

| | Phytoestrogens | | |
	Isoflavonoids	Lignans	Boron
Cauliflower		✓	✓
Celery root			✓
Chinese cabbage			✓
Corn			✓
Cucumbers	✓		✓
Dandelion leaves			✓
Eggplant	✓		
Endive			✓
Garlic	✓	✓	
Leeks		✓	
Lettuce, all types	✓		✓
Iceberg		✓	
Onions		✓	✓
Radishes			✓
Rutabagas			✓
Snow peas		✓	
Spinach			✓
Squash	✓	✓	
Sweet potatoes		✓	✓
Tomatoes	✓		✓
Turnips		✓	✓
Yams	✓		

4. *Try a boron-rich fruit salad.* Many of the fruits containing boron happen to be terrific when featured in a fresh fruit salad; try some combination of apples, bananas, berries (you can use unsweetened frozen varieties in the off-season), cantaloupe, and grapes. Toss a fruit salad together as often as you can. You can whip one up quickly by using an apple slicer, peeling and slicing a banana, and washing some grapes. To help prevent browning, remember to drizzle a vitamin C–rich fruit juice (such as orange juice, lemon juice, or grapefruit juice) over the top and toss. Store the fruit salad in an airtight container in the refrigerator, and voila! You and your family have refreshing fruit salad any time you want.

5. *Eat those year-round vegetables.* Several year-round vegetables, including broccoli, cabbage, carrots, and cauliflower, provide both phytoestrogens and boron. These vegetables are great to have on hand in your crisper or freezer (with the exception of cabbage, which doesn't defrost well) for a quick side dish for dinner. Just pop them in the microwave, and you've got vegetables for dinner in five minutes.

You can also eat broccoli, carrots, or cauliflower raw. Just wash and cut them into easy-to-handle sticks or stems. Keep the cut pieces covered in a little bit of water in a container in the refrigerator for convenience. Eat them as a cold, crisp, refreshing snack; dip them in a reduced-fat dressing or dip; or add them to salads or entrees such as pasta, rice dishes, or casseroles. Get them any way you can.

DIET COMMANDMENT #3:
Limit Your Intake of Caffeine, Soft Drinks, and Alcohol—and Drink Plenty of Water

This commandment, among other things, is about being kind to your kidneys by avoiding diuretics (substances that increase the release of urine) and by drinking lots of what the kidneys crave—water. This commandment may sound like no fun at all. But remember that it says to "limit" your intake of caffeine, soft drinks, and alcohol—not eliminate them from your life completely.

How to Drink 8 Cups of Water a Day

In order to get your 8 cups of water a day, you may need to "schedule" certain glasses of water into your routine. The trick is using certain daily activities as your cue to drink a glass of water (or other decaffeinated, nonalcoholic beverage). Perhaps start out the morning with a decaf latte made with nonfat milk, followed by orange juice blended with sparkling water. By midmorning, guzzle a glass of water. With lunch you might indulge yourself and have your one token can of caffeine-free cola. Come midafternoon, perhaps after going to the mailbox or some other daily cue, automatically drink another glass of water. If you're in the car running errands or going on a short trip, make sure to take along a sports bottle filled with water. About 30 minutes before your exercise class, drink a glass of water, and fill your sports bottle with more ice-cold water. With dinner drink a tall glass of ice water garnished with a wedge of lemon or lime. Later in the evening, either drink a cup of decaf herb tea or have another glass of water after brushing your teeth.

The point here is not to follow this hypothetical routine exactly, but to develop your own pattern cued by your own daily schedule. Altogether you might drink four to six large glasses of water and about three other decaffeinated beverages each day. And you'll want to pace your water consumption throughout the day so you don't feel as if you just swallowed a water balloon. You'll find that once you make drinking water a habit, preferably tied to your daily routine, you'll just do it without having to think about it so much anymore.

When You've Got to Have That Caffeine

Caffeine is a stimulant. If you really need a jump start in the morning, then do just that: Have your cup of caffeine (along with a balanced breakfast). But stop there. Caffeine isn't considered a drug by most experts because it can be discontinued without major discomforts. Some people can simply switch to decaffeinated alternatives, without much noticeable difficulty. Nor does caffeine consumption result in a craving for higher doses, as other drugs do. There is some evidence, however, that the majority of fairly heavy caffeine drinkers (those who drink the equivalent of 4 or more cups of coffee a day) will probably experience some caffeine withdrawal symptoms, the two most common being headaches and fatigue. The cure for this headache (and any other withdrawal symptoms) is simply to reduce your caffeine intake gradually rather than try to eliminate all your caffeine consumption overnight. Try reducing your caffeine quota by one cup every week until you're down to one or none.

Where Is Caffeine Lurking?
Caffeine can be found in tea, cocoa, chocolate, cola, alertness tablets, diuretics, cold and allergy remedies, as well as the notorious coffee beverages. Be sure to read labels carefully. (See exercise 3 of chapter 10 for guidelines on how to calculate the amount of caffeine in your diet.)

Limiting Your Intake of Soft Drinks
and Alcohol in the Real World

We rarely see vending machines at gas stations or in office buildings that offer bottles or cans of flavored waters or fruit juice. We can usually select only from colas or uncolas, caffeinated or decaffeinated (if we're lucky). And when you opt for fast food, your beverage choices are often various soft drinks, tea, coffee, milk shakes, or nonfat or low-fat milk (again, if you're lucky).

It takes a motivated person to rise above this predicament and drink lots of water and minimal soft drinks, alcohol, and caffeine. But menopause is a good time of life to be motivated. Holidays, parties, and sometimes even dinners or work meetings often revolve around alcohol and caffeine. Here are some tips if you want to keep your consumption of these beverages to a minimum. (Of course, if you have a serious problem with alcohol, please consider seeking professional help.)

- Order water with a slice of lemon or lime at fast-food restaurants.
- If you spend much time in your car, consider investing in a car refrigerator (or cooler) and stock it with all your favorite nonalcoholic, caffeine-free beverages.
- Pack a bottle of water in your car or purse at all times.
- When you go on day trips or to a party, bring your preferred beverage, be it mineral water, bottled water, nonalcoholic beer (there are some great ones available now), or decaffeinated iced tea.
- At parties or in bars and restaurants, order drinks that look like alcoholic beverages but aren't, such as:
  1. Club soda or sparkling water with a wedge of lemon or lime.
  2. Orange juice mixed with cranberry juice (with or without club soda or sparkling water).
  3. Tonic water without the gin but with a wedge of lime.
  4. A margarita or daiquiri without the liquor (virgin).
  5. A nonalcoholic beer.

DIET COMMANDMENT #4:
Eat about 150 Percent of the RDA for the Vitamins and Minerals You Need More of As You Age

This commandment refers specifically to vitamins B-6, B-12, D, and folic acid, and to the minerals chromium and zinc. (Calcium and the antioxidants are covered in Diet Commandments #6 and #7.) You can take a few simple steps to ensure that you are getting 150 percent of the RDA for these six nutrients. Table 9.2 lists the top food sources for them and indicates how much of each of these nutrients a typical serving of that food provides. And in the next text section, I'll suggest several foods that you can easily incorporate into your daily diet to provide most of these six important vitamins and minerals.

Ideas for Getting More of These Six Nutrients

Many of the foods that contain one or more of these six nutrients are foods we should be trying to work into our diet for other reasons anyway. Beans, for example, are good sources of phytoestrogens and fiber. But as Table 9.2

Table 9.2. Top Food Sources for Six Essential Vitamins and Minerals

Food Source and Serving Size	Vitamin B-6 (mg)	Folic Acid (µg)	Vitamin B-12 (µg)	Vitamin D (IU)	Chromium*	Zinc (mg)
	Nutrient Quantities Provided					
RDA for Adult Women	1.6	180	2.0	200 (5 µg)	†	12
Beans, Nuts, and Seeds						
Nuts in general					✓††	
Baked beans and similar, 1 cup						3.6
Black-eyed peas, cooked, ½ cup		120				
Garbanzo beans, canned, ½ cup		80				
Kidney beans, canned, 1 cup		126				
Lentils, cooked, ½ cup		180				
Miso (soybean product), ½ cup						4.6
Peanuts, ½ cup		106				
Pinto beans, cooked, 1 cup		294				
Refried beans, 1 cup						3.5
Sunflower seeds, ½ cup		141				
Cereals and Grains						
Whole grains in general					✓	
Brewer's yeast					✓	

*The precise amounts of chromium contained in various food servings were not available at the time of publication. However, chromium is known to be contained in the foods followed by a check mark in that column. The best known food sources of chromium are mushrooms, prunes, nuts, and asparagus. Other significant sources are meat, organ meats, whole grains, and cheese.

†There is not yet an RDA for chromium; however, 50–200 µg is generally considered safe and adequate.

††Information on specific nuts not available.

(continued next page)

Table 9.2.   (continued)

Food Source and Serving Size	Vitamin B-6 (mg)	Folic Acid (µg)	Vitamin B-12 (µg)	Vitamin D (IU)	Chromium*	Zinc (mg)
Maypo, ¾ cup	0.65					
Oatmeal, instant (all flavors), ¾ cup	0.77					
Cheese						
Cheese in general					✓†	
Frozen Desserts						
Frozen yogurt, average of all flavors, 1 cup			0.71			
Ice milk, regular, 1 cup			0.88			
Ice milk, soft-serve, 1 cup			1.40			
Fruits and Vegetables						
Artichoke, cooked		61				
Artichoke hearts, cooked, 3 oz		95				
Asparagus, cooked, ½ cup		88			✓	
Banana	0.66					
Boysenberries, 1 cup		84				
Broccoli, cooked, 1 cup		78				
Brussels sprouts, cooked, 1 cup		94				
Greens, cooked						
Collard, 1 cup		129				
Dandelion or turnip, 1 cup		82				
Lettuce						
Green leaf, fresh, 1 cup		60				

†Information on specific cheeses not available.

Table 9.2.   (continued)

Food Source and Serving Size	Vitamin B-6 (mg)	Folic Acid (µg)	Vitamin B-12 (µg)	Vitamin D (IU)	Chromium*	Zinc (mg)
Romaine, fresh, 1 cup		76				
Mushrooms					✓	
Orange juice, from concentrate, 1 cup		109				
Peas, 1 cup		100				
Potato, baked with skin	0.70					
Prunes, 3 dried	0.56					
Spinach, cooked from fresh, 1 cup		262				
Spinach leaves, fresh, chopped, 1 cup		109				
Winter squash, baked, 1 cup	0.50					
Meat †						
Meat in general, 3 oz					✓††	4.0
Ground beef, extra-lean, 3 oz			1.80			4.6
Lamb cutlet, cooked, 3 oz			2.20			
Lamb, leg of, lean only, 3 oz						4.2
Lamb, shoulder or rib roast, lean only, 3 oz						5.0
Round steak, lean only, broiled, 3 oz			2.50			4.0

†In consideration of space, only a select few of the many beef sources of vitamin B-12 are included.

††Information on specific meats not available.

(continued next page)

Table 9.2. (continued)

Food Source and Serving Size	Vitamin B-6 (mg)	Folic Acid (µg)	Vitamin B-12 (µg)	Vitamin D (IU)	Chromium*	Zinc (mg)
			Nutrient Quantities Provided			
Sirloin steak, lean only, broiled, 3 oz			1.70			4.4
Turkey, dark meat, 3 oz						3.8
Turkey ham, 2 oz			1.30			
Turkey pastrami, 2 oz			1.20			
Veal cutlet, broiled, 3 oz			1.40			4.3
Veal rib roast, 3 oz						3.8
Meat Dishes††						
Beef and vegetable stew, 1 cup			1.60			5.3
Beef and bean burrito			1.60			3.3
Beef burrito						5.8
Beef enchilada			1.00			
Chili with beans, 1 cup						5.1
Ham and swiss cheese sandwich on rye						3.0
Hamburger meat, 3 oz			0.78			4.0
Lasagna with meat, 1 serving			1.50			3.2
Meatloaf, beef only, 1 serving			1.90			3.5
Moussaka (lamb and eggplant), 1 cup						3.3
Patty melt on rye						6.6
Roast beef sandwich			1.50			3.7

†In consideration of space, only the most common meat dishes containing beef (as a source of vitamin B-12) are included.

Table 9.2. (continued)

Food Source and Serving Size	Vitamin B-6 (mg)	Folic Acid (µg)	Vitamin B-12 (µg)	Vitamin D (IU)	Chromium*	Zinc (mg)
Reuben sandwich						4.6
Spaghetti, with meat sauce, 1 cup			1.20			
Taco, beef			1.40			
Tostada with beef and beans			1.70			3.6
Tostada with chicken and beans			0.73			
Tuna noodle casserole, 1 cup			1.80			
Tuna salad sandwich			0.90			
Turkey sandwich			1.20			
Veal parmigiana, frozen entree						4.0
Milk						
Fortified milk in general, 1 cup				100		
Evaporated milk, canned, ½ cup				110		
Instant nonfat skim milk powder, ¼ cup			0.68			
Low-fat milk, 2%, 1 cup			0.89	100		
Nonfat milk, 1 cup			0.93	100		
Other Mixed Dishes						
Tostada with refried beans	1.00					
Seafood						
Bluefish, baked or broiled, 3.5 oz	0.53		7.10			
Bass, baked or broiled, 3.5 oz			3.40			

(*continued next page*)

Table 9.2. (continued)

Food Source and Serving Size	Vitamin B-6 (mg)	Folic Acid (µg)	Vitamin B-12 (µg)	Vitamin D (IU)	Chromium*	Zinc (mg)
Carp, baked or broiled, 3.5 oz			1.50			
Catfish, fried in cornmeal, 3.5 oz			2.00			
Clams, canned, 1 cup			158.00			4.4
Clams, steamed meat only, 20			89.00			
Cod, baked or broiled, 3.5 oz			1.10			
Cod liver oil, ½ tsp				110		
Crab, blue or Dungeness, 1 cup			10.00			5.5
Crab, imitation from surimi, 3 oz			1.40			
Eel, smoked, 1 oz				1,814		
Haddock, baked or broiled, 3 oz			1.20			
Herring, baked or broiled, 3.5 oz			13.00	892		
Lobster, cooked meat only, 1 cup			4.50			4.2
Mackerel, baked or broiled, 3.5 oz			19.00			
Manhattan clam chowder, 1 cup			7.90			
Mussels, blue, steamed, meat only, 3 oz	0.63		1.40			
Northern pike, baked or broiled, 3.5 oz			1.20			
Oysters, raw, 1 cup			40.00–48.00			40.0–224.0
Perch, baked or broiled, 3.5 oz			1.20			

Table 9.2.   (continued)

| | Nutrient Quantities Provided | | | | | |
Food Source and Serving Size	Vitamin B-6 (mg)	Folic Acid (µg)	Vitamin B-12 (µg)	Vitamin D (IU)	Chromium*	Zinc (mg)
Pollock, baked or broiled, 3.5 oz			3.10			
Rockfish, baked or broiled, 3.5 oz			3.20			
Salmon, baked or broiled, 3 oz			4.90			
Salmon, pink, canned, 3.5 oz			4.6	284		
Sardines, canned, 3.5 oz			9.00	297		
Scallops, steamed, 3.5 oz			1.90			
Sea trout (steelhead), cooked, 3.5 oz	0.8		5.7			
Shrimp, boiled, 3.5 oz			1.50			
Shrimp, canned, 3 oz			0.9	90		
Snapper, baked or broiled, 3.5 oz			1.60			
Sole, baked or broiled, 3 oz			2.10			
Swordfish and trout, baked, 3 oz			2.00			
Tuna, light, packed in water, canned, 6 oz	0.62		5.60			
Yogurt						
Low-fat yogurt, plain, 1 cup			1.30			
Low-fat yogurt, with fruit, 1 cup			1.10			
Nonfat yogurt, 1 cup			1.40			

shows, beans also contribute folic acid, zinc, and vitamin B-6. Nonfat or low-fat milk is a great source of calcium. But drinking just a cup a day also helps us get vitamins D and B-12. Eating more dark green leafy and cabbage-family (cruciferous) vegetables is a great idea because they contain important antioxidants and phytochemicals. But eating dark green leafy vegetables will also contribute folic acid, while the cabbage-family vegetables will contribute some vitamin B-6.

Here are some more foods (or supplements) that contribute at least two of these six important nutrients:

- *Canned tuna*, light, packed in water, will contribute vitamins B-6 and B-12 (as will bluefish and blue mussels).
- A serving of *lean beef* will contribute vitamin B-12, zinc, and chromium.
- A serving of *beans* will contribute folic acid, and some zinc, and small amounts of vitamin B-6 (too small to be listed in the table).
- Switching to *whole-grain products* when possible—for your cold and hot cereals, bread, and so on—will contribute some chromium and zinc.
- Drinking a serving of *nonfat or low-fat milk* a day (or eating items made with milk, like puddings or pancakes) will contribute both vitamins D and B-12.
- Taking one of the *vitamin-mineral supplements* listed in Table 5.2 will contribute 100 percent of the RDA for vitamin D, folic acid, vitamins B-6 and B-12, and zinc, as well as approximately 25 micrograms of chromium (half the minimum estimated safe and adequate amount, which is 50 to 200 µg).

DIET COMMANDMENT #5:
Eat Many Small Meals throughout the Day, and Eat Light at Night

Eating many small meals throughout the day doesn't mean that you still eat a big lunch and a big dinner and just add snacks in between. It means that instead of eating a big breakfast, with cereal, toast, coffee, and juice, you might have toast and coffee first thing, then have cereal and juice later that morning. It means that you divide your usual lunch into two small meals, which you eat maybe 2 to 3 hours apart. And it means that instead of eating a large dinner, you opt for a nice midafternoon snack and a light dinner. This type of schedule works out great for all you postwork exercisers: If you're going to work out between work and dinner, the midafternoon snack should supply you with plenty of energy during your workout.

Barriers to Eating Light—and What to Do about Them

Following this Diet Commandment can be difficult for many of us. Here are several of the barriers in place in modern life, along with suggestions for overcoming them.

Barrier #1: It's Not Socially Acceptable

It's simply not socially acceptable to eat many small meals throughout the day and to eat light at night. If you eat a snack about 10:30 A.M., people say something like, "Boy, I wish I could eat as many meals as you do," or, "You're going to ruin your lunch." But if "ruin" means you're not going to eat a large meal, then, by all means, go ahead—ruin your lunch, and ruin your dinner, too. Because avoiding large meals, especially large dinners, is a good thing.

Barrier #2: Work Schedules

Our work schedules tend to reinforce the no-holds-barred lunch. Most 9-to-5ers work straight through their morning until finally they surface to take a lunch at noon or 1 P.M., when they're way past the point of reasonable hunger. Force yourself to take a midmorning break. It's a good time to fix yourself a bowl of microwave oatmeal, or to have a fruit salad, or a bagel with light cream cheese. If you do, you are more likely to be satisfied with a lighter lunch later. By midafternoon, you might be ready for a salad, some microwave low-fat popcorn, or low-fat yogurt with low-fat granola.

Barrier #3: Family-Style Dining

Family traditions tend to promote the concept of large dinners—and don't forget that nice rich dessert at the end of the big meal. Traditionally, dinner is the meal when the family comes together. Decades ago this was the meal that the wife/mother spent her afternoon preparing, and this was the meal the man of the house anticipated coming home to after a longs day's work. Sorry to spoil the image of June Cleaver in the kitchen, but when you eat large meals like this late in the day, you're likely to end up in an easy chair, dozing off in front of the evening news. You're not going to burn many calories in this reclined position, nor afterward lying in bed.

Even some diet drink commercials encourage dieters to drink their very low cal shakes for breakfast and lunch and then have a "sensible meal" for dinner. Metabolically speaking, if we drink those very low cal shakes at all, it should probably be at dinner—not breakfast or lunch, when our energy demands are highest.

I don't mean to discourage family mealtimes; eating dinner together isn't the problem. But the size and composition of the traditional evening meal usually is. You might want to try eating dessert earlier that day, perhaps as an afternoon treat. Or how about dishing up a dessert that's smaller in size? To help you retrain yourself to eat light at night, try using salad plates instead of the larger dinner plates for your evening meals. If you're really hungry, go ahead and have seconds. However, if you're not really hungry but you want seconds anyway, make yourself a plate and wrap it up for lunch tomorrow.

If you think about it, family dinners actually promote lighter eating because they encourage lots of conversation. When you talk, you eat more slowly, giving your body a chance to feel full and eat less.

How to Eat Light

This commandment and these mealtime tips are not about low-calorie dieting or depriving yourself of food if you're hungry. They're about restructuring your meals, rearranging when you consume your calories, to promote high energy, and to meet your metabolic needs more efficiently so as to discourage extra body fat from accumulating over time. Probably the best advice is to listen to your body. Let its natural hunger rhythms guide you. If you eat a low-fat, moderately sized lunch, you're likely to be hungry for a midafternoon snack. Make the switch from satisfying your eyes and traditional meal expectations to satisfying your physical hunger. One additional benefit of eating light at night is that you're more likely to wake feeling invigorated, with an appetite the size of Texas. So give it a chance. See how it feels to eat many smaller meals and snacks throughout the day and to eat light at night.

˙DIET COMMANDMENT #6:
Eat at Least Two Calcium-Rich Foods Every Day, Preferably Ones Also High in Vitamin D

Drinking milk and consuming other dairy products are probably the quickest ways to make a big dent toward getting the 1,500 milligrams of calcium recommended for postmenopausal women who are not on HRT or ERT (or the 1,000 mg recommended for women who are taking estrogen). Not only does a cup of milk provide about 245 milligrams of calcium, it also delivers it to you in the fine company of vitamin D and lactose, two strong calcium-absorption enhancers. That's wonderful news if you're a milk-drinker. But many people are not milk drinkers, either because they don't like the taste, or because they're lactose-intolerant, or perhaps because they don't want the calories that milk provides—which water, iced tea, and diet soft drinks don't.

If you don't like the taste of milk, try adding chocolate syrup. This really isn't as bad for you as it sounds. Chocolate syrup, while contributing sugar, is virtually fat-free, made mainly of cocoa and sweetener. Or learn to appreciate the simple pleasure of a good decaf latte (or cappuccino), in which espresso coffee is mixed with steamed milk. Especially if you use nonfat or low-fat milk, these flavorful beverages can be good daily sources of calcium.

If you're lactose-intolerant, you're going to have to consume nondairy sources of calcium (see Tables 7.1 and 9.3 for some detailed lists). But if calories and fat are your concern, then the answer is to consume nonfat or low-fat milk and dairy products. In most cases, nonfat milk has even more calcium than regular milk. The same advantage is held by low-fat or fat-free yogurt over regular varieties. This truth always seems to surprise people. A popular myth exists that as you decrease the fat in your diet, you'll get fewer nutrients. In fact, the main difference between a high-fat diet and a low-fat diet is fat! If anything, in the case of most water-soluble vitamins and most minerals, you actually get more, not less, on a low-fat diet and by making leaner, lower-fat choices.

Calcium-Rich Foods to Choose From

Everybody has his or her own personal list of food likes and dislikes. So Diet Commandment #6 is going to mean different things to different people. For example, a milk drinker would probably make a point of working in a couple of servings of nonfat or low-fat milk, perhaps as a beverage or as an ingredient in a breakfast shake. On the other hand, someone who isn't a milk drinker may decide to eat some nonfat or low-fat yogurt on days when she isn't getting any reduced-fat cheese. Table 9.3 offers a list of foods rich in calcium and shows which of these are also rich in vitamin D and/or magnesium. Use this table to find the foods you like, looking particularly for ones that contain vitamin D and/or magnesium. Decide which ones you wouldn't mind having every day—or every other day. You may want to circle these or jot them down as a reminder. For more practical tips on how to get more calcium in your diet, read on.

Milk—Tops in Calcium, Vitamin D, and Magnesium

What's the quickest way to get a dose of calcium and two other calcium-absorption enhancers, without a lot of extra fat or calories? Drink a glass of lower-fat *milk*. Milk beats other calcium-rich foods hands down when it comes to the amount of calcium provided and the presence of two important calcium-absorption enhancers, vitamin D and lactose. And as long as you select nonfat or 1% low-fat milk, you can get your calcium with next to no fat. But what can you do if you're not a milk drinker? The answer is that there are ways of consuming milk without drinking it plain.

Table 9.3. Calcium-Rich Foods (Which May Also Be Rich in Vitamin D and Magnesium)

Food Serving	Nutrient Contents Provided*		
	Calcium (mg)	Vitamin D	Magnesium
Black-eyed peas, boiled, 1 cup	212		
Broccoli cooked with reduced-fat cheese sauce, 1 cup	298		
Cheese			
Low-fat cheddar or colby, 1 oz	199		
Low-fat mozzarella, 1 oz	207		
Low-fat swiss, 1 oz	272		
Parmesan or romano, 1 oz	301–335		
Cocoa mix, sugar-free, unfortified, 1 small packet	216		M
Cocoa mix with calcium, Alba, sugar-free, 1 packet	327		M
Evaporated 2% low-fat milk, 4 oz	358	D	M
Evaporated nonfat milk, canned, 4 oz	370	D	M
Frozen yogurt, low-fat, 1 cup	300		M
Frozen yogurt, nonfat, 1 cup	325		M
Greens			
Collard, boiled from frozen, 1 cup	358		M
Turnip, boiled from fresh, 1 cup	250		M
Ice milk, premium (Breyer's Light), 1 cup	216		
Milk			
2% low-fat milk, 8 oz	298	D	M
1% low-fat, 8 oz	300	D	M
1% low-fat milk with calcium, 8 oz	550	D	M
1% lactose-reduced low-fat milk, 8 oz	302	D	M
Buttermilk, nonfat, 8 oz	284		M
Chocolate milk, 2% low-fat, 8 oz	285	D	M
Chocolate milk, 1% low-fat, 8 oz	288	D	M
Chocolate milk, nonfat, 8 oz	292	D	M
1% lactose-reduced low-fat milk with calcium, 8 oz	550	D	M

*D indicates that the listed food serving provides at least 20 IU of vitamin D; M indicates that the listed food serving provides at least 30 mg of magnesium.

Table 9.3.   (continued)

	Nutrient Contents Provided*		
Food Serving	**Calcium (mg)**	**Vitamin D**	**Magnesium**
Nonfat milk, 8 oz	301	D	M
Nonfat dry milk powder, 1 oz	349	D	M
Potatoes au gratin, homemade, 1 cup	292		M
Pudding, chocolate, made with 2% low-fat milk, 1 cup	306		M
Pudding, rice mix, made with 2% low-fat milk, 1 cup	302		M
Pudding, tapioca, made with 2% low-fat milk, 1 cup	298		M
Pudding, vanilla, made with 2% low-fat milk, 1 cup	292		M
Shake mix with calcium (Alba, chocolate), 8 oz	203		M
Spinach, boiled from frozen, 1 cup	278		M
Tofu, firm, ½ cup	258		M
Yogurt			
Low-fat fruit yogurt, 1 cup	345		M
Low-fat yogurt, flavored, 1 cup	388		M
Low-fat yogurt, plain, 1 cup	415		M
Nonfat fruit yogurt with low-cal sweetener, 1 cup	369		M
Nonfat yogurt, flavored, 1 cup	403		M
Nonfat yogurt, plain, 1 cup	451		M

Working Milk into Your Day

Try any or all of the following:

- Make your oatmeal with milk instead of water. You can add milk when
- making instant oatmeal too.
- Order a decaf latte made with nonfat milk.
- If you're craving chocolate, mix some chocolate syrup (virtually fat-free) in nonfat milk for a tasty treat.

- Have cream soups more often; just make them with nonfat or 1% low-fat milk. This approach can work with canned cream soups, too; just buy the new lower-fat cream soups on the market. Or you can add nonfat or 1% low-fat milk to a can of regular tomato soup to make a creamy tomato soup.
- Make low-fat shakes by blending nonfat or 1% low-fat milk with fruit, low-fat yogurt, or low- or nonfat frozen yogurts or ice milks.
- If you like an occasional diet-type shake as a snack or quick meal (the ones fortified with vitamins and minerals), blend it up with nonfat milk.

Working Other Calcium-Rich Dairy Foods into Your Day

Say Cheese

Cheese is a virtual staple for many Americans. And why wouldn't it be? Most of our favorite foods are loaded with it: pizza, macaroni and cheese (though not from a box since the packaged types use powdered cheese sauce), and lasagna, to name a few. And many of our favorite sandwiches feature a slice or two of cheese. There are so many great-tasting lower-fat cheeses available that we would do ourselves a favor to switch over to them, not only to consume less calories from fat but also to get more calcium. For reduced-fat cheeses actually provide *more* calcium per serving than the high-fat ones.

Yell for Yogurt

Nonfat and low-fat varieties of yogurt used to be the exception; now they're the norm. Today you'd be hard-pressed to find a carton of full-fat yogurt. And there are all sorts of interesting flavors now, too, such as strawberry-kiwi, cappuccino, or apricot-mango. The old standbys of lemon and vanilla are, fortunately, still available as well. Yogurt makes a great snack: It comes in its own convenient container, it has a nice balance of protein and carbohydrates, and it offers just about the right amount of calories for a snack. It also makes a good dressing for fruit salad. And yogurt can be substituted for mayonnaise in salad dressings and dips. You can also use yogurt (instead of frozen yogurt or ice cream) as the base for your breakfast or other fruit shake.

Add a little fun to your yogurt:

- Swirl in low-fat granola or low-fat muesli cereal.
- Sprinkle in raisins or other dried fruit.
- Stir fresh fruit, like raspberries or blueberries, into plain, lemon, or vanilla yogurt.
- Make a yogurt dessert by adding chocolate teddy grahams to your cappuccino yogurt, or mix your yogurt with light Cool Whip and make a parfait by sprinkling in layers of graham cracker crumbs.

- Add a touch of cinnamon to low-fat vanilla yogurt to make a delicious dip for fruit.

Working Calcium-Rich Plant Foods into Your Day

Dairy products aren't the only food sources of calcium. There are plenty of plant foods that contain a healthy amount of calcium, too. Here are the top plant sources of calcium (see also Table 9.3) and some tips to help you get more of them.

1. *Collard, turnip, beet, and dandelion greens.* Start looking for low-fat recipes that call for greens. You might want to try southern-style cookbooks.
2. *Frozen or cooked spinach.* Add spinach to soups, casseroles, lasagna, and so on, whenever possible.
3. *Tofu.* See the section titled "Tofu Mania," later in this chapter.
4. *Black-eyed peas.* In your favorite recipes, substitute black-eyed peas for other beans that are not as rich in calcium. Black-eyed peas also make a great side dish for fish, Mexican, and southern-style entrees.
5. *Kale.* Add kale to stir-fry recipes, casseroles, and soups, or eat it as a vegetable side dish.
6. *Bok choy.* Add bok choy to stir-fry recipes, casseroles, and soups, or eat it as a vegetable side dish.
7. *Baked beans.* Baked beans make a great side dish, especially in winter.
8. *White, navy, great northern, and kidney beans.* Add beans to casseroles, soups, and green or pasta salads. Eat bean salads more often. Look for low-fat bean recipes in southwestern and vegetarian cookbooks.
9. *Spinach leaves, fresh.* Make green salads with all or some spinach leaves.
10. *Broccoli.* Add broccoli to hot and cold pasta dishes, soups, casseroles, and stir-fry recipes. Broccoli also makes a great side dish for lunch or dinner.

DIET COMMANDMENT #7:
Eat Several Antioxidant-Rich Foods Every Day

While scientists scramble to uncover the mysteries of which antioxidants hold which disease prevention properties, the commonsense advice is to take in about two to three times the RDA of each. Eating two to three times the RDA of vitamin C and beta-carotene is a piece of cake: All you have to do is drink a 10-ounce glass of orange juice and eat a carrot every day. And if you don't like orange juice or carrots, there are plenty of other foods high in vitamin C and beta-carotene to choose from. On the other hand, getting enough (fat-soluble) vitamin E could be difficult if you're limiting the fat in your diet—unless you happen to like eating lima beans, soybeans, tofu, kale, or sweet potatoes (the only low-fat foods that are rich in vitamin E). You may want to take a supplement.

I have interviewed a dozen researchers across the country about vitamin E, and while many of them couldn't make a formal statement supporting vitamin E supplements, quite a few of them were presently supplementing their own diets with 200 to 400 IU of vitamin E.

Table 9.4 lists food servings that provide at least 50 percent of the RDA of one of the three main antioxidants—beta-carotene (a precursor of vitamin A), vitamin C, and vitamin E.

DIET COMMANDMENT #8:
Eat No More Than 20 to 25 Percent of Your Calories from Fat

If you eat a typical American diet right now, you're probably getting about 35 percent of your calories from fat. Lowering your fat intake from 35 percent to around 20 percent is going to require a few major changes, so take a deep breath. We're going to look first at where the majority of fat is coming from in the typical American diet, and then methodically identify quick and painless ways to trim it. We should, however, be able to eat healthily without giving up many of our favorite foods. After all, food should be enjoyed, not put up with. Recipes should be delicious, not acceptable. And we should feel satisfied, not deprived, after a meal. Our goal, therefore, will be to consume less fat without compromising any of these quality-of-life objectives.

Where's the Fat?

Here are the top 15 sources of fat in the typical American woman's diet, and simple steps you can take to eat less of each of them. (This information, published in the *Journal of the American Dietetic Association,* comes from a survey analysis of consumption data for women of all incomes aged 19 to 50, conducted by Dr. Krebs-Smith, Ph.D., R.D., with the National Cancer Institute.)

1. *Salad dressings* contribute 9.2 percent of the fat in a typical American woman's diet. To cut fat here, you can buy or make reduced-fat salad dressings. Read the labels, and look for a salad dressing with 3 grams of fat or less per tablespoon. (Recipes for quick, homemade reduced-fat dressings are provided in appendix B.)

2. *Margarine* contributes 7.9 percent of the fat in a typical American woman's diet. Buy the best-tasting diet margarines for spreading on bread or waffles, making garlic bread, and so on. Look for diet margarines with 2 grams of fat per teaspoon, such as I Can't Believe It's Not Butter Light.

Table 9.4. Antioxidant-Rich Foods

Food Serving	Antioxidants Provided*		
	Beta-Carotene	Vitamin C	Vitamin E
Fruits			
Cantaloupe, cubed, 1 cup	✓	✓✓	
Grapefruit, half		✓	
Grapefruit sections, canned, ½ cup		✓	
Guava, half		✓✓	
Kiwi		✓✓	
Mango	✓✓	✓✓	
Mango slices, ½ cup	✓	✓	
Orange		✓✓	
Orange sections, fresh, ½cup		✓	
Papaya, half		✓✓	
Papaya slices, ½ cup		✓	
Strawberries, whole or sliced, ½ cup		✓	
Tangelo		✓	
Tangerine sections, ½ cup		✓	
Vegetables			
Beet greens, boiled, 1 cup	✓	✓✓	
Bell pepper, red, half		✓✓	
Bell pepper, yellow, half		✓✓	
Bell pepper, red, chopped, ½ cup		✓✓	
Broccoflower, steamed, 1 cup		✓✓	
Broccoli pieces, cooked, 1 cup		✓✓	
Broccoli pieces, raw, 1 cup		✓✓	
Brussels sprouts, boiled, 1 cup		✓✓	
Butternut squash, baked and mashed, ½ cup	✓✓		
Butternut squash, baked cubes, 1 cup	✓✓	✓	
Carrot	✓✓		

*Those food servings that provide at least 50 percent of the RDA for a given antioxidant are followed by a check mark in that column. Those food servings that provide around 100 percent of the RDA for a given antioxidant are followed by two check marks in that column.

(*continued next page*)

Table 9.4.   (continued)

Food Serving	Antioxidants Provided*		
	Beta-Carotene	Vitamin C	Vitamin E
Carrot, raw, grated, ¼ cup	✓		
Carrot slices, steamed, ½ cup	✓✓		
Cauliflower, boiled, 1 cup		✓✓	
Cauliflower, raw, 1 cup		✓✓	
Chicory greens, raw, chopped, 1 cup	✓		
Chili peppers, raw or canned, ¼ cup	✓	✓✓	
Chinese cabbage, steamed, 1 cup		✓✓	
Dandelion greens, boiled, 1 cup	✓✓		
Dandelion greens, raw, 1 cup	✓		
Dock/sorrel greens, raw, chopped, 1 cup	✓	✓✓	
Green pea pods, cooked, 1 cup		✓✓	✓
Hubbard squash, baked cubes, 1 cup	✓✓		
Hubbard squash, boiled and mashed, ½ cup	✓		
Kale, boiled, 1 cup	✓✓	✓✓	✓
Kohlrabi, boiled, 1 cup		✓✓	
Lamb's-quarters, boiled, ½ cup	✓✓		
Mustard greens, boiled, 1 cup	✓	✓	
Peas, raw, 1 cup		✓✓	
Peas and carrots, boiled, 1 cup	✓✓		
Pumpkin, boiled from fresh, ½ cup	✓✓		
Pumpkin/squash mix, canned, ½ cup	✓✓		
Snow peas, steamed, 1 cup		✓✓	
Spinach, boiled, 1 cup	✓✓		
Spinach, fresh, chopped, 2 cups	✓	✓	
Sweet potato, baked without skin	✓✓		✓
Sweet potatoes, canned, ½ cup	✓✓		✓
Swiss chard, boiled, 1 cup	✓	✓	
Turnip greens, boiled, 1 cup	✓✓	✓	
Winter squash, baked cubes, 1 cup, or mashed, ½ cup	✓		
Yams, orange, mashed, ½ cup	✓✓		

Table 9.4. (continued)

	Antioxidants Provided*		
Food Serving	Beta-Carotene	Vitamin C	Vitamin E
Fruit and Vegetable Juices			
Apple juice (plus vitamin C), 8 oz		✓✓	
Cranberry juice cocktail, low-cal or regular, 8 oz		✓✓	
Grapefruit juice, 8 oz		✓✓	
Orange juice, 8 oz		✓✓	
Pineapple juice, 10 oz		✓	
Pineapple juice (plus vitamin C), 8 oz		✓✓	
Strawberry juice, 8 oz		✓✓	
V-8, low-sodium or regular, 8 oz		✓✓	
Yellow passion fruit juice, 8 oz			
Beans and Bean Products			
Lima beans, cooked from dry, 1 cup			✓
Soybeans, cooked from dry, 1 cup			✓✓
Tofu, ½ cup			✓
Nuts and Nut Butters			
Almonds, 1 oz			✓✓
Almond butter, 2 Tbsp			✓
Filberts/hazelnuts, 1 oz			✓
Soybeans, roasted, ½ cup			✓
Sunflower seed butter, 2 Tbsp			✓✓
Sunflower seed kernels, roasted, 2 Tbsp			✓✓
Oils			
Almond oil, 1 Tbsp			✓
Cottonseed oil, 1 Tbsp			✓
Hazelnut oil, 1 Tbsp			✓
Rice bran oil, 1 Tbsp			✓
Safflower oil, 1 Tbsp			✓
Sunflower oil, 1 Tbsp			✓✓
Other			
Mayonnaise, 1 Tbsp			✓

3. *Cheese* contributes 7.6 percent of the fat in a typical American woman's diet. Buy the best-tasting reduced-fat cheeses, such as Cracker Barrel Light Sharp Cheddar, Kraft ⅓ less fat singles, and Kraft Reduced Fat block cheeses. And use fat-free or light cream cheese.

4. *Ground beef* contributes 6.7 percent of the fat in a typical American woman's diet. Buy ground sirloin or ground beef that is around 10 percent fat. If you're so inclined, you can blend ground sirloin with a lower-fat tofu or ground turkey breast product. Of course, you can always use all ground turkey breast (although it is going to look and taste altogether different from ground beef).

5. *Luncheon meats and sausages* contribute 5.4 percent of the fat in a typical American woman's diet. Buy the lunch meats that are lean (around 98 percent fat-free). Buy the lower-fat sausages (including low-fat turkey sausage products) and the lower-fat hot dogs, which are 85 percent fat-free or better.

6. *Beef cuts* contribute 5 percent of the fat in a typical American woman's diet. Choose leaner cuts of beef, and use cooking methods that use very little fat while producing a tender, tasty dish.

7. *Whole milk and whole-milk beverages* contribute 4.5 percent of the fat in a typical American woman's diet. Switch to lower-fat or nonfat milk. Order your coffee drinks or tea with nonfat or low-fat milk.

8. *French fries, potato chips, and other fried potatoes* contribute 4.1 percent of the fat in a typical American woman's diet. Buy lower-fat frozen french fries and bake instead of fry them. Buy lower-fat frozen hashbrowns, and pan-fry them with two-thirds less fat, or use chicken broth and no fat. Buy reduced-fat potato chips, or eat naturally low-fat pretzels instead.

9. *Poultry* contributes 4 percent of the fat in a typical American woman's diet. Buy chicken breasts rather than dark meat when possible. Take the skin off all chicken pieces before or after cooking. And cook poultry with very little or no added fat.

10. *Vegetable shortening* contributes 3.9 percent of the fat in a typical American woman's diet. Remember, shortening is 100 percent fat. So use the least amount possible, and consider adding something lower in fat instead.

11. *Eggs* contribute 3.8 percent of the fat in a typical American woman's diet. The fat and cholesterol are in the yolk. So using egg whites is fine. Use fewer whole eggs in baked recipes. (You can usually get by with one whole egg and some fat-free egg substitute.) In egg dishes such as omelettes and quiche, try using half real eggs and half fat-free egg substitute.

12. *Pork* contributes 3.7 percent of the fat in a typical American woman's diet. Pork, in general, is much leaner than it used to be. There are many fairly lean cuts available today, but the tenderloin is by far the leanest. Add very little or no fat when cooking pork. Trim visible fat before cooking.

13. *Butter* contributes 3 percent of the fat in a typical American woman's diet. Butter tastes so good, you can usually get by with using a lot less than you're used to. When making cookies, brownies, cakes, or biscuits, you can usually cut the amount of butter *in half.* Add another low-fat ingredient instead (try applesauce, light sour cream, flavored yogurts, or fat-free cream cheese).

14. *Cooking oils* contribute 2.7 percent of the fat in a typical American woman's diet. Use as little oil as possible. Rely on nonstick cooking sprays and ingredients that can serve as replacements for some or all of the fat. Instead of deep-frying foods, bake or grill them. Instead of pan-frying or stir-frying foods, simmer or stir-fry them in fat-free liquid like broth, wine, beer, or fruit juice.

15. *Salty snacks, crackers, and tortillas* contribute 2.4 percent of the fat in a typical American woman's diet. Buy reduced-fat crackers and snack foods when possible. Read the labels, and look for products with 3 grams of fat or less per ounce of crackers or chips. Many of the classic crackers now have 50 percent less fat versions. There are several reduced-fat, great-tasting potato chips available now, too. Try Ruffles or Pringles Light or Mr. Phipps Tater Crisps.

As a group, the various fats and oils together (margarine, vegetable shortening, butter, and cooking oils) contribute a total of 18 percent of the fat in a typical American woman's diet. The fat contributed by the fried potato group (french fries, potato chips, and other fried potatoes) comes primarily from cooking fat, adding another 4 percent to the fats and oils total. And if you add the fat contributed by the number-one category, salad dressings, where the majority of the fat probably comes from oil, the combined total for fats and oils climbs to over 30 percent of all the fat in a typical American woman's diet.

The combined total from ground beef and other beef cuts is 12 percent of the fat in a typical American woman's diet. The importance of trimming meat of visible fat becomes clear when you realize that, based on this survey analysis, when trimmed and untrimmed beef are grouped separately, the trimmed beef supplies 8 percent of the protein, 5 percent of the iron, and only 2 percent of the fat in a typical American woman's diet, while the untrimmed beef supplies only 3 percent of the protein, only 2 percent of the iron, yet 3 percent of the fat.

What about Saturated Fat?

It stands to reason that if you reduce the amount of total fat in your diet, you will most likely reduce the amount of saturated fat as well, especially if you're eating less fat from animal sources and more plant foods in general.

But we can still learn a lot by analyzing where most of our saturated fat is coming from. So here are the top 10 sources of saturated fat for American women of all incomes aged 19 to 50, along with the percent of the total that each provides:

1. Cheese: 13.4 percent.
2. Ground beef: 7.8 percent.
3. Whole milk and whole-milk beverages: 7.8 percent.
4. Beef cuts: 5.6 percent.
5. Luncheon meats and sausages: 5.6 percent.
6. Butter: 5.1 percent.
7. Margarine: 4.2 percent.
8. Salad dressings: 4.2 percent.
9. Ice cream and other frozen dairy desserts: 3.9 percent.
10. French fries, potato chips, and other fried potatoes: 3.7 percent.

Beef cuts combined with ground beef contribute a total of 13.4 percent of all saturated fat, enough to put them in a tie for first place with cheese. Butter and margarine, if grouped together, would rise to second place, contributing a total of 9.3 percent of all saturated fat.

Since many of us are used to eating meat and/or have meat-loving families, let's now turn our attention to how to find and prepare leaner meats.

Cooking Leaner Meat

Lean meats can easily be part of a healthful, low-fat diet. The keys are to choose the leanest meats, trim away any visible fat, prepare them with the least amount of added fat, and serve them in moderate-sized portions (3 to 4 oz of cooked meat, about the size of a deck of playing cards). Those suggestions may not sound like much fun, but they can be. Many of our favorite dishes—Chinese food, chili con carne, spaghetti, and shish kebabs—already incorporate them.

Beef

The leanest beef cuts are:

- Eye of round (roast or steak).
- Round tip (kebab).
- Top loin (New York, club, or strip steak).
- Tenderloin (filet mignon, fillet steak).
- Sirloin (sirloin steak, London broil).
- Top round (London broil).

All have 8 grams of fat or less and 80 milligrams of cholesterol or less per 3-ounce portion, cooked and trimmed.

Ground Beef

The leanest type of ground beef available is usually ground sirloin (approximately 13 percent fat by weight). Ground sirloin usually contains around 170 calories, 7 grams of fat, and 65 milligrams of cholesterol per 3-ounce cooked portion.

Pork

The leanest pork cuts (in order) are:

- Tenderloin, with 133 calories, 4 grams of fat, and 67 milligrams of cholesterol per 3-ounce cooked portion.
- Boneless sirloin chops.
- Boneless loin roasts.
- Top loin chops.
- Center loin chops.

Sirloin roasts, boneless rib roasts, and rib chops have 175 to 179 calories, 8.5 to 8.8 grams of fat, and 69 to 73 milligrams of cholesterol per 3-ounce lean, cooked portion.

Lamb

The leg shank and the sirloin center loin chops are the two leanest lamb cuts. They both contain less than 185 calories and 8 grams of fat or less per 3-ounce cooked portion.

Chicken and Turkey

Skinless chicken and turkey breast are your best meat choices when it comes to fat. One skinless chicken breast (3 oz) contains only 141 calories, 3 grams of fat, and 73 milligrams of cholesterol. One 3-ounce portion of turkey breast contains only 119 calories and 1 gram of fat. And if you remove the skin from chicken or turkey thighs, those servings are still lower in fat than many other types of meat (around 150 calories and 6 g of fat per 3-oz serving).

Finding Low-Fat Meat Products

Is there such thing as a healthful hot dog? Is bacon ever healthy? Lunch meats and sausages contribute over 5 percent of the fat in the average woman's diet. But there are so many low-fat lunch meats and reduced-fat cured-meat products now available that bringing this percentage down a few points should be fairly easy. The following sections offer some tips on how to do so. But remember, because these products are processed and/or preserved, they will likely contain from 200 to 400 milligrams of sodium per ounce.

Cold Cuts

Look for products that contain 2 grams of fat or less per ounce. Healthy Choice isn't the only brand that offers a multitude of choices; so do Butterball Deli Thin, Foster Farms, Hillshire Farm Deli Select, Louis Rich Deli Thin, Louis Rich Carving Board, Mr. Turkey Deli Cuts, and Oscar Mayer Deli Thin.

Bologna

Attention bologna lovers: Louis Rich now makes a 50 percent less fat turkey bologna, and Oscar Mayer makes a beef bologna with half the fat of their regular bologna.

Bacon

Louis Rich, Turkey Selects, and Butterball all make a turkey bacon that contains 50 percent less fat than regular bacon (approximately 5 g of fat per two strips).

Hot Dogs

If you want a reduced-fat hot dog that tastes like it still has all the fat, try the hot dogs with 50 percent less fat (around 6 g of fat per frank). There are quite a few brands that make hot dogs with only 1 gram of fat, but you may not like the way they taste.

Sausages

There are a few light sausage breakfast links on the market, containing from 5 to 11 grams of fat per two links. Louis Rich, Healthy Choice, and Hisshire Farm offer at least two reduced-fat large sausages each with only 4 grams of fat per cooked ounce.

Vegetarian Diets

Many vegetarians think that they are eating low-fat diets simply because they avoid meat. Unfortunately, that's not always the case. Nuts and seeds, oil, all-vegetable shortening, peanut butter, and cheese are common ingredients in meatless recipes. These ingredients have one thing in common: fat. Indeed, a vegetarian's diet can qualify as a high-fat diet just as easily as an omnivore's can. Simply getting rid of meat doesn't get rid of all the fat in your diet.

Finding Other Lower-Fat Products in the Supermarket

Here are some tips, for vegetarians and omnivores alike, for reducing the fat contents of foods other than meat.

Salad Dressings
Salad dressings contributed the highest percentage of fat in women's diets, probably for two reasons: (1) We pour a ton of dressing on our salads, and (2) our favorite dressings are very high in fat. However, reduced-fat alternatives now occupy a large portion of the salad dressing shelf. Look for dressings that contain no more than 5 grams of fat and no more than 500 milligrams of sodium per 1-ounce serving (2 Tbsp).

Mayonnaise
Look for mayonnaise that contains no more than 5 grams of fat per tablespoon. There are several fat-free mayonnaises on the market, but not everyone is going to like the way they taste.

Cheese
Cheese is the third-largest fat contributor in the average American woman's diet. The quickest way to lower fat in this category is to switch to reduced-fat cheeses and use a little less each time you have cheese. There are many great-tasting cheeses with 3 to 5 grams of fat per ounce; look for them. There are also fat-free cheeses—though, again, you may not like the way they taste. However, you might want to try mixing them with cheeses that have 5 grams of fat per ounce.

Cream Cheese
There are several reduced-fat cream cheeses available, including Philadelphia Free, which makes a good fat substitute in some recipes, and Philadelphia Light (in the tub), which goes well on bagels and whatnot.

Favorite Light Products
There are hundreds of light products to choose from in the supermarket today. One of the easiest ways to reduce fat in your diet is simply to substitute nonfat, reduced-fat, and/or light products whenever possible. See which reduced-fat products you and your family like, then stick with those. Here are some possibilities to consider:

- Light Best Foods Mayonnaise.
- Bernsteins Light Fantastico Salad Dressings.
- Cracker Barrel Light Sharp Cheddar Cheese.
- Louis Rich 50% Less Fat Turkey Bacon.
- Louis Rich 50% Less Fat Turkey Hot Dogs.
- Jones 50% Less Fat Sausage & Rice Links.
- Ritz Reduced Fat Crackers.
- Pringles and Ruffles Light Potato Chips.
- Snack Well's Reduced Fat Creme Sandwich Cookies.

- Philadelphia Light Cream Cheese (as a spread).
- Philadelphia Free Cream Cheese (as a fat substitute in some recipes).
- Dreyer's and Breyer's Light Ice Cream.
- I Can't Believe It's Not Butter, Light (diet margarine).
- Campbell's Healthy Request Soups.
- Land O'Lakes Light Sour Cream.
- Classico Onion and Garlic Spaghetti Sauce.

Remember, you always have choices. When buying canned or packaged foods like cereals, crackers, soups, and frozen entrees, choose products that have the least amount of fat. Take the time to read the nutrition information label; you only have to look at it once to know whether it's lower in fat or not. Compare it to the regular-fat products to see how much lower in fat it truly is. Also check the sodium and calories; perhaps they added more sugar and sodium in the lower-fat version (they sometimes do, to compensate for the taste loss). And check the serving sizes: Are they realistic?

Cook Right—Cook Light!

The road to cooking light is really a five-step program.

1. *Use cooking techniques that do not require fat.* Try grilling, simmering, baking, poaching, steaming, broiling, roasting and smoking whenever possible.
2. *Don't follow the directions.* Don't be afraid to add less fat than the directions on the package or in the recipe call for. In most cases, you can cut the amount of added butter, margarine, or oil in half and add a replacement (or substitute). With some products you don't have to add *any* of the fat called for; this applies to cake mixes (though be sure to add a fat replacement, such as light sour cream, maple syrup, nonfat cream cheese, or applesauce, to compensate for the fat not added), pancake mixes, frozen french fries, frozen pot stickers, puddings, and salad dressing packets.
3. *Know how low you can go.* The amount of fat that can be successfully cut out of a recipe depends on that particular recipe. With cookies, for example, you can usually only cut the fat in half. However, the fat in cakes can sometimes be cut down to $\frac{1}{4}$ cup, while in muffin recipes the fat can be cut to 2 tablespoons of oil or butter per 12-muffin batch. Experiment by cutting the butter, margarine, shortening, or oil in half (that's usually a good place to start)—then see how the recipe turns out and fine-tune the reduction from there.
4. *Know your fat replacements.* When you take fat out of a recipe, you generally have to add something back in to give it the moisture, the flavor, and the right consistency. Certain fat replacements tend to work best in certain

recipes. Specifically, try using light or fat-free sour cream as a fat replacement in brownies and chocolate desserts, fat-free cream cheese as a fat replacement in cookie recipes, fruit purees like applesauce or crushed pineapple in spice or carrot cakes or muffins, liqueur as a fat replacement in dessert recipes, and wine as a fat replacement in stove-top and stir-fry recipes. Don't be afraid to experiment to find your own favorite fat replacements.

5. *Give it time.* Experts are now finding that when fat is reduced gradually in the diet, fat cravings are more likely to be held at bay, and that when a low-fat diet is followed regularly, a person's taste preference for fat drops eventually. So be patient, and work on lowering your fat consumption day by day, a little at a time.

Where Do We Go from Here?

I hope this book is only the beginning to your learning about low-fat cooking and eating. Seek out pamphlets that list lower-fat products, read books that focus on low-fat cooking and eating, and cut out recipes that satisfy this Diet Commandment. And, of course, I recommend my other books on low-fat cooking. I've written several and am sure to do more since lightening up recipes has become my passion.

DIET COMMANDMENT #9:
Eat 20 to 30 Grams of Fiber Every Day, from a Variety of Different Foods

We need a variety of fiber in our diet. Soluble fiber, found in oats, beans, and many fruits and vegetables, is thought to help lower both cholesterol and triglyceride levels in the blood. Wheat fiber, on the other hand, is credited as being the best at providing bulk in the large intestines, helping exercise the muscles in the intestinal wall, and moving food waste through the intestines quickly and effortlessly.

When some people start eating more fiber, they experience a bit of discomfort, such as gas and uncomfortable intestinal blockages. Try a few of the following steps to minimize these discomforts:

- Increase your fiber consumption gradually.
- Eat well-balanced meals slowly; chew your food thoroughly.
- Drink more liquids (water especially) as you increase your fiber consumption.

To increase your total fiber consumption, switch to whole-grain breads whenever possible, eat at least five servings of fruits and vegetables every day, eat beans more often, and eat a high-fiber cereal every day as part of your breakfast or as a snack. Table 10.3 (in the next chapter) lists the fiber content of a great many foods.

Eat a High-Fiber Cereal

By switching to a high-fiber breakfast cereal, adding crunchy high-fiber cereal to your yogurt, or having high-fiber cereal as a snack, you can increase your daily fiber intake by at least 4 grams with each serving. Look for a cereal that contains at least 4 grams of fiber per serving, provides 25 percent or less calories from fat, and 25 percent or less calories from sugar if it doesn't contain dried fruit. If the cereal contains dried fruit, then look for 30 percent or less calories from sugar (the natural sugar from the dried fruit is calculated in the sugar total). Look also for cereal with less than 400 milligrams of sodium per serving. To help you select from the multitude of breakfast cereals on the market, see Table A.4 in appendix A.

DIET COMMANDMENT #10:
Moderate Your Intake of Sodium and Sugar

The goal here is to *moderate* your consumption of sodium and sugar, not *eliminate* them from your diet completely. It's easy to point the finger at dietary foes and say absolutely that they're bad. But the truth often isn't that simple—as with sodium and sugar. Our bodies need a little sodium, an electrolyte, to survive, and our taste buds expect a little sweetness to be satisfied. So where do we draw the line? The body actually needs way less sodium than even the amount recommended on a low-sodium diet—around 2,000 to 2,400 milligrams a day. However, this level of sodium is, in most cases, low enough to achieve the health benefits desired. Unlike sodium, however, our bodies don't *need* refined sugar. But sweetness certainly is a pleasurable taste experience, and sugar exists in many popular foods. In fact, we are born with a preference for sweet-tasting substances. Diabetics strive to eliminate simple sugars altogether, but the rest of us can certainly have moderate amounts without any major health repercussions.

How to Curb Your Sugar Intake

First, do you know where the sugar in your diet is coming from? Nine to 13 percent of the calories in the average adult diet come from refined sweeteners, most of them in processed foods. Soft drinks are the single biggest source, responsible for about 21 percent of our refined sugar intake. We get 18 percent of our sugar from the sweet group (including syrups, jellies and jams, gelatin desserts, ices, popsicles, and table sugar itself), while 13 percent comes from the baked dessert category (including cakes, cookies, pies, pastries, and sweet crackers). Adding these three groups together accounts for over half of our sugar consumption. What about that downfall of many of us, ice cream? Another 10 percent of our sugar consumption comes from milk products, including ice cream, puddings, and yogurts, and 6 percent from breads and grains. A surprising 5 percent comes from breakfast cereals.

When you look at these percentages, you can see that for many people, the best, most painless way to limit sugar consumption is to avoid sweetened soft drinks. If you really enjoy your sodas, you don't have to abandon them completely. Cut down to one token soft drink a day, or switch to diet soda— but even then you should still have only one a day, because of the phosphorus content in carbonated beverages and because you're better off drinking water or a beverage with nutrients. If keeping soda in the house will make you drink more than one a day, reserve your token sodas for when you go out.

Besides cutting sweetened sodas, here are some other ways to reduce your sugar intake:

1. Buy jams, syrups, gelatin desserts, popsicles, and so on, with the least amount of added sugars when possible. (See Table A.5 in appendix A for specific suggestions.)
2. Avoid adding sugar to foods at the table.
3. Let yourself eat cake—and cookies, ice cream, or candy. But be reasonable. Perhaps limit yourself to one such goodie a day. This way you aren't depriving yourself to the point where you develop strong cravings or binge.
4. Read the labels on packaged foods. The standard nutrition label format usually combines starches and sugar into one carbohydrate category. But some product categories, like cereals, are labeling sugar seperately. Keep in mind, though, that often the natural sugars from dried fruit (like raisins) are combined in this total.
5. Avoid heavily sugared cereals (again, read the labels carefully).
6. Use artificially sweetened diet products in reasonable amounts. Be aware, though, that some sugar-free products in large amounts (like sorbitol) can cause diarrhea and intestinal discomfort.

Lightening Up on Sodium and Salt

Unlike with sugar, we are not born with a preference for sodium or salt. But we do seem to develop a taste for it in our food. Once you lower the sodium in your diet, food may temporarily taste bland. However, a couple months later (or less) your taste threshold for sodium starts to readjust to the lower level, and the former, higher level will seem distastefully salty.

Sources of Sodium

Probably the biggest contributor to our total sodium intake is salt. Salt is made up of sodium and chloride (NaCl). One teaspoon of salt contains almost 2,000 milligrams of sodium. Other sodium sources are the flavor enhancer **monosodium glutamate** (MSG, found in the product Ac'cent) with 492 milligrams of sodium in 1 teaspoon, **sodium nitrite** (used in cured meats and sausages), **sodium benzoate** (a preservative in condiments like relishes, sauces, and salad dressings), and soy sauce. There are also natural amounts of sodium found in meat, fish, poultry, eggs, milk, and milk products. However, since most of our sodium comes from the salt added to food during commercial processing and home preparation, you're best off paying less attention to the amounts of natural sodium in your food and more attention to the sodium you and food companies add to it.

Start Cutting Sodium at the Table

Based on USDA consumption surveys conducted from 1989 through 1991, women over the age of 50 take in approximately 2,400 milligrams of sodium daily, not including any extra salt or sodium added at the table or during the cooking. So, since you're already close to the maximum of 2,400 milligrams of sodium a day *without* any extra salt added at the table, probably the most logical place to cut your sodium intake is at the table.

Tips for Cutting Sodium at the Table

1. Take the salt shaker off the table and put it into a cabinet. You're much less likely to use it if it isn't right in front of you.
2. Ask yourself whether you even taste your food before you salt it. Some of us get into the habit of shaking something on our food—and that's hard to stop. Maybe all you need is a substitute seasoning to shake, like pepper, Italian herb seasoning, or a salt-free seasoning blend.
3. Make a deal with yourself to try at least 6 weeks of lower-sodium cuisine before you go back to salting your food. It takes about that long for your taste buds to adjust to the lower level of sodium. After about 6 weeks, formerly bland-tasting (lower-sodium) items should taste better to you.
4. If there are just a couple of foods you absolutely must shake salt on—such as french fries, popcorn, or maybe watermelon—then at least make sure you sprinkle rather than pour it on. You can even shake the salt into the palm of your hand, then add it, pinch by pinch, to your food.

Tips for Cutting Sodium in the Kitchen

Salt is an important ingredient in most baked recipes, such as muffins, cookies, and cakes. It adds flavor, is part of the leavening, and helps control yeast growth in yeast breads. So you really don't want to cut the sodium in these recipes. Also the amount of sodium in these recipes usually ends up being relatively little per serving. On the other hand, with foods like scrambled eggs, chicken, and tuna casserole, that are made for two to four people, any added teaspoon of salt quickly starts building up your sodium intake. Avoid adding other sodium sources to recipes, too, like monosodium glutamate (Ac'cent) and soy sauce. Instead, add other flavorings that don't contain a lot of sodium, such as fresh herbs, fresh garlic, ginger and other seasoning aids, salt-free seasoning blends, freshly ground pepper, or a touch of Tabasco sauce.

Tips for Cutting Sodium in the Supermarket

Here is where it can get a bit confusing. In a few product categories, it seems as if you need to choose between moderating your sodium and moderating your fat. There are reduced-sodium cheeses that are not reduced-fat. There are reduced-sodium crackers that are not reduced-fat. And there are reduced-fat cheeses and crackers that are not reduced-sodium. When in doubt, buy the reduced-fat product unless your doctor has advised you specifically to buy the reduced-sodium product. The difference in sodium between many of the reduced-fat crackers and the low-salt version of the same crackers is only about 75 to 150 milligrams per serving.

Remember that the most important steps are not adding salt or other sources of sodium at the table and while cooking. If you can comfortably cut sodium by buying lower-sodium products, great. But always opt for the reduced-fat products first. And sometimes, as is the case with fat-free Mister Salty Pretzels, they are lower in fat *and* lower in salt.

Here are some other ways to cut some sodium in the supermarket:

1. Read the right label. Don't worry about finding all the sodium sources in the ingredients list. The nutrition label will tell you how much sodium there is per serving.
2. Choose from three brands of lower-fat, lower-sodium soups: Healthy Request Campbell's Soup, Healthy Choice Soups, and Progresso Healthy Classics Soups. Generally the sodium is cut by a third or half. (Table 9.5 compares the sodium, fat, and calorie contents of three varieties of these three brands of light soups.)
3. Buy no-salt-added or low-sodium canned vegetables and canned tomato products when possible. Tomato puree and tomato paste tend to contain less added sodium than tomato sauce.

Table 9.5. Comparing the Light Soups

Soup Varieties and Brands	Each 1-Cup Serving Provides		
	Fat (g)	Sodium (mg)	Calories
Chicken Noodle			
Healthy Request (Campbell's)	3.0	480	160
Progresso Healthy Classics	2.0	480	80
Healthy Choice	2.0	460	130
New England Clam Chowder			
Healthy Request (Campbell's)	3.0	480	110
Progresso Healthy Classics	2.0	530	120
Healthy Choice	1.5	480	120
Minestrone			
Healthy Request (Campbell's)	2.0	480	120
Progresso Healthy Classics	2.5	510	120
Healthy Choice	1.5	470	110

4. Limit your use of foods bottled in brine (salt water), like pickles, sauerkraut, and olives. When you do use them, drain the salt water and rinse the food well before adding it to the dish.

5. Moderate your consumption of hot dogs, smoked meats, sausage, ham, bacon, luncheon meat, and canned or processed fish. These cured and processed products tend to be high in sodium.

6. Buy lower-sodium soy sauce and teriyaki sauce.

7. Buy fresh garlic and onion or garlic and onion powder instead of garlic salt, onion salt, or seasoning salt.

8. When using salt-containing meat tenderizers or marinade products, use half as much tenderizer or marinade powder with the same amount of liquid (and use beer, wine, or lemon or pineapple juice instead of water for more flavor) to cut the sodium in half.

9. Buy lower-sodium broth or broth packets for recipes.

10. Buy lower-sodium chips and crackers when they are also lower in fat.

11. Choose the low-fat frozen entrees with no more than 800 milligrams of sodium per serving. In general, the amount of sodium in the health-oriented brands of frozen dinners (Weight Watchers, Lean Cuisine, Healthy Choice, and so on) have come down substantially over the past few years. There are a lot more lower-fat, lower-sodium entrees to choose from today.

12. When you buy fairly high sodium products like bottled spaghetti sauce or catsup, realize that you will not need to add any sodium in the cooking or on the table.

13. Don't spend your sodium all in one place, such as with many fast-food choices. Lower-fat fast-food options, such as grilled chicken breasts or bean burritos, may also be lower in sodium.

14. Avoid buying higher-sodium beverages. Check the labels, and avoid those with over 40 milligrams per 12 ounces. The top offenders are tomato juice, 360 milligrams per 6 ounces (unsalted tomato juice contains just 5 mg per 6 ounces); and V-8 vegetable juice, 980 milligrams per 6 ounces (Light & Tangy V-8 contains 75 percent less sodium, just 240 mg per 6 ounces).

FOLLOWING SEVERAL DIET COMMANDMENTS AT ONCE

You can meet the standards of at least half of the 10 Diet Commandments simultaneously by following three general strategies:

1. Eat more beans.
2. Eat more tofu or soybeans.
3. Eat more fruits and vegetables.

The remainder of this chapter will discuss the hows and whys of these three basic guidelines.

Beans: The Wonder Food

You can follow five of the 10 Diet Commandments just by doing one thing—eating beans. This may seem hard at first—diet surveys have shown that the average person typically gets only 6 to 7 percent of his or her fiber from beans and legumes, one of the highest-fiber foods around. But there are many benefits to adding more to our diets.

The Benefits of Beans

- Beans appear to slow the absorption of glucose into the bloodstream. Thus, they might curb your appetite longer. (They may also cause your body to need less insulin, a major benefit for diabetics.)
- Total blood cholesterol tends to *decrease* significantly while the ratio of HDL (good) cholesterol to LDL (bad) cholesterol *increases* significantly on a diet rich in bean fiber.
- Beans are packed with fiber.

- Soybeans contain isoflavones, a kind of phytoestrogens. Lentils, soybeans, kidney beans, navy beans, pinto and fava beans are rich in lignans, another kind of phytoestrogen.
- Beans contain other beneficial phytochemicals as well, including protease inhibitors, phytosterols, and saponins.
- Beans are a low-fat source of protein.
- Beans are great sources of many vitamins and minerals we might need more of as we age, like folic acid and vitamin B-6.

Table 9.6 lists your best bets for beans—those varieties that are highest in eight key nutrients. This table also indicates which varieties are known sources of two kinds of phytoestrogens, lignans and isoflavonoids. The beans included in the table are listed in descending order based on which varieties provide the highest quantities of the key nutrients listed. As you can see from the table, many popular varieties of beans—including soybeans, lentils, navy beans, kidney beans, and others—are excellent sources of protein, fiber, and many important vitamins, minerals, and phytochemicals.

The First Major Barrier to Eating Beans

There are two sugars that occur naturally in beans, **raffinose** and **stachyose,** that can produce certain side effects like flatulence and gastrointestinal distress, because we don't have an enzyme needed to digest them. But the extent to which this affects you depends on how much gas-producing bacteria you have in your intestines. So if you're committed to eating beans but have experienced some discomforts or embarrassments because of them, there are several things you can do:

- Add beans to your diet slowly. Eat no more than $\frac{1}{2}$ cup per day about twice a week to start.
- If you soak your beans before cooking them, replace the soaking water with fresh water to cook them.
- "Beano" is a product that contains the enzymes that break down the gas-producing sugars in beans. Manufacturer suggestions advise you to add a few drops only to the first bite of your bean serving.

The Second Major Barrier to Eating Beans

Besides the gas barrier, people also avoid beans because they don't have the time or inclination to soak, rinse, boil, and drain the dried beans. But if you are in too much of a hurry to hassle with all this, you are buying your beans in the wrong supermarket aisle. Try the canned-vegetable section the next time you're in the market for beans. All you need is a can opener and about 20 seconds, and boom—you'll have more beans, ready-to-eat, than you'll know what to do with. The taste and variety of canned beans have improved considerably in the past few years. Of course, the sodium content is going to be higher in canned beans. However, for some brands it will be only 200 milligrams per $\frac{1}{2}$ cup serving (S&W 50% Less Salt or Progresso).

The Third Major Barrier to Eating Beans

Now we know to buy canned beans for convenience (preferably the varieties canned without salt or with less salt). What's the next barrier? Many of us don't know how many good ways there are to eat beans. To learn, we can look to other cultures, since many ethnic cuisines depend on the bountiful bean for their protein and complex carbohydrates. And we can become creative, adding beans anywhere possible. Here are some ideas:

- Add beans to soups, stews, chili, or sloppy joes.
- Add beans instead of, or in addition to, meat in Mexican dishes.
- Toss a few beans together with a light Italian dressing for a quick side dish.
- Sprinkle some beans on your green salad, chicken, or taco salad.
- Serve bean dips at parties, or keep them in the refrigerator for a quick snack.
- Try the bean recipes included in appendix B.

Tofu Mania

Eating soybeans and soybean products like tofu helps us to meet Diet Commandments #1 and #6. There are still some uncertainties, but it appears that soybeans are one of those special "wonder foods" God put on this earth, like garlic and broccoli. Here are some of the health advantages to eating soybeans and soybean products like tofu:

- Soybeans and tofu contain phytoestrogens (isoflavones) that act like estrogen when absorbed into the body.
- Soybeans contain other phytochemicals, besides phytoestrogens, that help protect our bodies against cancer. (They may even contain several more protective-type substances that we don't even know about yet.)
- Soybeans and tofu are rich in calcium.
- There is some scientific evidence that soy protein (particularly if it replaces animal protein in your diet) can lower your LDL (bad) cholesterol level, and that the isoflavonoids in soybeans seem to prevent and reduce the formation of plaque—fatty deposits on artery walls.

Americans eat an average of only 3 pounds of soy foods per person per year; the Japanese eat 24 pounds. A recent study, published in the *American Journal of Clinical Nutrition,* compared Chinese and Japanese people who ate tofu and soybeans on a regular basis with people from the midwestern United States who ate virtually no tofu. Researchers concluded that the lower

Table 9.6. The Best Beans

Type of Bean	Protein (g)	Fiber (g)	Folic Acid (mg)	Calcium (mg)	Iron (mg)	Zinc (mg)	Magnesium (mg)	Vitamin B-6 (mg)	Source of Lignan	Source of Isoflavonoid
Beans with six nutrient amounts in the top five										
Soybean	28.6	6.0	93	175	8.8	2.0	147	0.40	✔	✔
Beans with five nutrient amounts in the top five										
Lentils	17.9	10.0	358	38	6.6	2.5	71	0.35	✔	
Beans with four nutrient amounts in the top five										
Navy beans	15.8	16.0	255	127	4.5	1.9	107	0.30	✔	
Winged	18.3	0.9	18	244	7.5	2.5	93	0.08		
Beans with three nutrient amounts in the top five										
Baby lima	11.6	16.0	45	54	4.2	1.3	125	0.30		
White beans	16.1	14.1	245	130	5.1	2.0	121	0.23		
Black beans	15.2	15.4	256	46	3.6	1.9	120	0.12		
Pinto beans	14.0	19.5	294	82	4.5	1.0	94	0.27	✔	

Beans with two nutrient amounts in the top five

Kidney beans	15.3	15.0	229	50	5.2	1.9	80	0.20
Black-eyed peas	5.2	12.2	356	211	1.9	1.7	86	0.11
Garbanzo beans (chick peas)	14.5	11.1	282	80	4.7	2.5	79	0.23

Beans with one nutrient amount in the top five

Great Northern	14.7	10.7	181	120	3.8	1.6	89	0.20
Large lima	11.9	16.5	156	51	4.4	1.6	94	0.20
Green peas	8.6	7.7	50	43	2.5	1.9	62	0.35
Yardlong beans	14.2	2.8	249	72	4.5	1.9	167	0.16

All amounts shown are per 1 cup, cooked.

mortality rates from breast and prostate cancer of Japanese women and men, respectively, may be due to their high intake of soybean products.

What Is Tofu, Exactly?

Tofu is made by filtering cooked, pureed soybeans. The "milk" that forms is curdled using coagulants. The whey is drained off and the curds are pressed into blocks—that's tofu. Because tofu is relatively low in calories and high in water content, the percentage of calories from fat appears to be high, but per serving, tofu is actually a fairly low-fat food. The grams of fat per 4-ounce serving can range from 2 to 5 grams. And more than half the fat is polyunsaturated.

How to Use Tofu

There are two ways to use tofu: (1) as a featured ingredient, as it is in Chinese and Japanese cuisine, or (2) as a fat replacement or meat extender (because it is rather colorless and neutral-tasting). In the case of the latter, you will generally get the best results if you puree the bean curd then blend it with another ingredient. Tofu has little flavor of its own so it picks up flavors nicely from other ingredients added to it. For example, tofu hamburgers, which are made by combining ground sirloin with tofu, honestly look and taste like they're 100 percent beef. The only noticeable difference is that the tofu hamburgers are more moist and tender (not necessarily a negative change).

Here are some tips for buying, keeping, and using tofu:

- Check the expiration date on your package of tofu before you buy it, and open the package only when you are absolutely ready to use it. Cover any unused tofu with water, cover the container, and refrigerate it. Remember to change the water at least every other day; if you don't, the tofu can go bad rather quickly.
- If you freeze tofu for a few days, after you thaw it out it will crumble into pieces—a quality that might be desirable when using tofu in certain recipes.
- Mix tofu, half and half with the original higher-fat ingredient (usually meat or cheese). If you eliminate the original ingredient altogether and replace it completely with tofu, you will get an entirely different dish—one you and your family may not like.
- Use tofu as an extender when the texture and taste of tofu won't interfere with the aesthetics of the dish, or the qualities that make that dish special.
- You can marinate and grill or broil tofu in the same sauces you would chicken or beef.
- Add tofu to your stir-fry recipes in place of, or in addition to, meat.

- Tofu is an excellent featured ingredient in its own right. Chinese and Japanese cuisines have enjoyed this prized soybean curd for hundreds of years. Experiment with Asian recipes that use tofu. (For several recipes using tofu, check appendix B.)

Other Ways to Eat Soybeans

In Asia, they eating other soy-based foods in addition to tofu. One popular variation is **tempeh,** a chewy cake of soybeans often mixed with rice or millet. It is described as having a smoky or nutty flavor, and it can be steamed, marinated, and then grilled. It can also be added to mixtures like spaghetti sauce or chili. A second option is **miso,** a salty condiment that blends soybeans, and sometimes a grain, with salt. Miso is used to flavor soups, sauces, and marinades. Soup stock can be made blending $\frac{1}{4}$ cup of miso with 4 cups of water. Miso is high in sodium, however, so it should be used sparingly.

There are also many manufactured soy products available in the west. You might consider trying fat-free, all-soy franks, soy-based breakfast sausages, soy breakfast entrees, or soy burgers. However, when you are checking soy and other vegetarian products offered in your supermarket, don't forget to read the nutrition labels to note the amount of fat per serving, and the ingredient labels to see whether soybeans are a major ingredient.

Eat 5-a-Day: It's the Sure Way

Along with eating beans and tofu, another way to satisfy several Diet Commandments at once is to eat at least five servings of fruits and vegetables a day. This is actually easier than it sounds. It's also more important than was previously thought many years ago when the "5-a-Day" program was first conceived by the California Department of Health Services. Why? Because getting your five fruits and vegetables each day can help you get:

1. Phytoestrogens (Diet Commandment #1), since many fruits and vegetables provide phytoestrogens.
2. Boron (Diet Commandment #2), since many fruits and vegetables contain boron.
3. At least 150 percent of the RDA of many of the vitamins and minerals that we need more of as we age (Diet Commandment #4).
4. More calcium in your diet (Diet Commandment #6), if you select dark green leafy vegetables as one of your five servings.
5. More antioxidants (Diet Commandment #7), since many fruits and vegetables are the best sources of vitamin C and beta-carotene, two of the three most important antioxidants.
6. A lower-fat diet (Diet Commandment #8), since fruits and vegetables are naturally low in fat (with a few exceptions, such as coconut, olives, and avocados).

7. More fiber (Diet Commandment #9), since most fruits and vegetables are super sources of fiber.

8. Less sodium and sugar (Diet Commandment #10), since most *fresh* fruits and vegetables are naturally low in sodium and sugar. (Fruits frozen or canned *without* added sugar, and vegetables frozen or canned *without* added salt are also available in most supermarkets.)

Why Five?

Five servings of fruits and vegetables was the magical number that appeared to be strongly protective against cancer in most of 200 epidemiological studies recently reviewed by Gladys Block, a renowned researcher. Also, the people who though it up no doubt thought "5-a-Day" had a nice ring to it. And believe it or not, five servings of fruits and vegetables a day seems to be enough of a challenge for many people. Indeed, results from a national survey showed that less than a tenth (9 percent) of the people in the United States ate five servings of fruits and vegetables a day (*Journal of the National Cancer Institute*).

How to Eat More Fruits and Vegetables

How do you eat more fruits and vegetables? The answer is the Nike slogan, "Just Do It!" Most of us know we should eat more fruits and vegetables. Most of us probably even *want* to eat more fruits and vegetables. But do we? Nope. Why not? For many of us, it may be a combination of habit and convenience. Most of our convenience-food sources (fast foods, pizza parlors, frozen foods) don't provide a large variety of fruits and vegetables to choose from. Nor are they providing large portions of fruits and vegetables, if any at all. And whether it's true or not, most people think it's easier to open a box of crackers or a bag of chips or cookies than to grab an apple, peel an orange, open a can of soup, or toss up a small salad. Beyond that, many of us just aren't in the habit of having fruits and vegetables with every meal and as snacks.

So here are some tips to make eating fruits and vegetables more convenient, and more of a habit:

- Pack your work desk or car with your favorite dried fruits (dried apricots, dried prunes with essence of lemon or orange, raisins, or a dried fruit medley).
- Stock your refrigerator with your favorite 100 percent fruit juices. Maybe even buy individual servings so you can grab them while you're running out the door.
- Take time Sunday or at the beginning or end of the work week to make a large spinach salad, or vegetable fortified lettuce salad, so you'll have

salad ready at your whim for at least 3 days (store it in an airtight container, and don't put dressing on until you're ready to eat it).

- Do the same with a fresh fruit salad. Drizzle lemon juice or other citrus juice over the top, and toss to coat the fruit with it (the vitamin C helps prevent browning). Store the fruit salad in an airtight container in the refrigerator so that it will be available to have with breakfast, lunch, dinner, or as a snack without any further fuss. (Great fruit salad fruits are seedless grapes, canned pineapple chunks packed in pineapple juice, kiwi slices, bananas, orange sections, canned mandarin oranges, melon cubes or balls, and whole strawberries.)
- Start each morning with a glass of fruit juice.
- Eat a certain fruit (or fruits) every morning with breakfast or as a morning snack, like half a grapefruit, canned or fresh peaches, or half a cup of fresh or frozen berries.
- If you like juice smoothies, create interesting fruit and/or vegetable juice combinations, and drink one every day as you would a vitamin-mineral supplement or medicine.
- Almost always have a mixed green salad (including vegetables like tomatoes, carrots, broccoli florets, and green peppers) or a spinach salad with lunch or dinner.
- Eat a raw carrot (or other raw, fresh vegetable like celery, broccoli, or cauliflower) at about the same time every day—perhaps while making dinner.

Following the 10 Diet Commandments will most likely require a few shifts in your present eating practices. But hopefully the tips in this chapter will make it fairly painless. And if you find yourself slipping back into a less healthful way of eating—you can always return to the 10 Diet Commandments, and this chapter, and set yourself on the right path again. The key is incorporating some of these ideas and tips into your everyday life and making them *habits*—healthy ones to last a lifetime.

10

MONITORING YOUR PROGRESS

To figure out how far you still have to go to follow the 10 Diet Commandments, you need to know where you are right now. The most accurate way to analyze your present diet is with a computer program that tracks everything you eat in a day, perhaps for several days. A Registered Dietitian can also perform that service for you, usually for about $100. (If you would like a referral, call the American Dietetic Association Consumer Hotline at 800–877–1600.) If the software and expert options are not available, or not to your taste, this chapter can help.

Start by writing down what you eat during a 24-hour period in the "1-Day Food Record." Then go through the exercises in this chapter, which help you measure your current diet against each individual Diet Commandment. You'll also find in this chapter tables listing foods relevant to particular Diet Commandments, and the amount(s) of the nutrient(s) they contain. For example, you could count up how much fiber you ate yesterday by looking through Table 10.3, marking the high-fiber foods you ate, and adding up the total grams of fiber you consumed.

You can complete a 1-Day Food Record as many times as you like. Just make a photocopy of this page from the book each time you want to fill one out. It's up to you whether you want to see how you measure up on a typical or a good day. Of course, you can always do both—all it will cost you is a little more of your time.

1-Day Food Record   Day: M Tu W Th F Sat Sun

Time of Day	Food or Drink Consumed	Amount	Calories	Fat (g)	Protein (g)	Sodium (mg)	Fiber (g)

Now add up your totals
for the final five columns.   Total   Total   Total   Total   Total

EXERCISE #1   Are You Eating at Least One Phytoestrogen-Rich Food Every Day?

DIET COMMANDMENT #1
Eat at Least One Phytoestrogen-Rich Food Every Day

Compare the foods listed in your 1-Day Food Record with the lists of foods rich in lignans and isoflavonoids (see Tables 9.1, A.1, and A.2). If you've had at least one serving of a food from any one of these lists, make a note of which food(s) you had and whether they were high in lignans or isoflavonoids (or both).

Foods I ate that are rich in phytoestrogens:

	Food	Lignans	Isoflavonoids
Examples:	broccoli	✓	✓
	pear	✓	

1. _____ rich in _____   _____

2. _____ rich in _____   _____

3. _____ rich in _____   _____

4. _____ rich in _____   _____

5. _____ rich in _____   _____

EXERCISE #2   Are You Eating at Least One Boron-Rich Food Every Day?

DIET COMMANDMENT #2
Eat at Least One Boron-Rich Rich Food Every Day

Compare the foods listed in your 1-Day Food Record with the lists of boron-rich foods (see Tables 9.1 and A.3). If you've had at least one serving, make a note of all the boron-rich foods you had.

Foods I ate that are rich in boron:

1. _____

2. _____

3. _____

4. _____

5. _____

EXERCISE #3   How Much Caffeine and Soda Are You Really Drinking?

DIET COMMANDMENT #3
Limit Your Intake of Caffeine, Soft Drinks, and Alcohol—and Drink Plenty of Water

Step 1
Review your 1-Day Food Record to determine if any of the items listed below were consumed. If so, note how many servings of each you had in the next-to-last column.

Step 2

Calculate what your soda and caffeine totals were for the day, using the chart below.

Calculating Your Caffeine Consumption

Beverage/Food	Serving Size (oz)	Average Caffeine Content (mg)		Number of Servings per Day		Total Caffeine Content (mg)
Coffee, Tea, and Chocolate						
Roasted and ground coffee (percolated)	5	74	×	_____	=	_____
Roasted and ground coffee (drip)	5	112	×	_____	=	_____
Instant coffee	5	66	×	_____	=	_____
Roasted and ground coffee, decaffeinated	5	2	×	_____	=	_____
Instant coffee, decaffeinated	5	3	×	_____	=	_____
Tea (hot or iced)	5	27	×	_____	=	_____
Instant tea (hot or iced)	5	28	×	_____	=	_____
Hot cocoa	5	4	×	_____	=	_____
Milk chocolate	1	6	×	_____	=	_____
Chocolate milk	8	5	×	_____	=	_____
Soft Drinks						
Regular colas	12	up to 46	×	_____	=	_____
Diet colas	12	up to 58	×	_____	=	_____
Decaffeinated colas	12	trace	×	_____	=	_____
Decaffeinated diet colas	12	trace	×	_____	=	_____
Now add up the two totals indicated.				_____ Total		_____ Total

EXERCISE #4   Are You Getting about 150 Percent of the RDA of the Nutrients You Need More of As You Age?

DIET COMMANDMENT #4
Eat About 150 Percent of the RDA for the Vitamins and Minerals You Need More of As You Age

---

Answer the following questions, referring to your 1-Day Food Record:

1.   Did you take a complete vitamin-mineral supplement, one that provides 100 percent of the RDA for vitamin B-6, folic acid, vitamin B-12, vitamin D, and zinc, and that provides at least 25 µg of chromium?   Yes or No

2.   Did you eat at least one of the foods listed in Table 9.2 as being a good source of vitamin B-6?   Yes or No

How many different servings of such foods did you have?   _____

3.   Did you eat at least one of the foods listed in Table 9.2 as being a good source of folic acid?   Yes or No

How many different servings of such foods did you have?   _____

4.   Did you eat at least one of the foods listed in Table 9.2 as being a good source of vitamin B-12?   Yes or No

How many different servings of such foods did you have?   _____

5.   Did you eat at least one of the foods listed in Table 9.2 as being a good source of vitamin D?   Yes or No

How many different servings of such foods did you have?   _____

6.   Did you eat at least one of the foods listed in Table 9.2 as being a source of chromium?   Yes or No

How many different servings of such foods did you have?   _____

7.   Did you eat at least one of the foods listed in Table 9.2 as being a good source of zinc?   Yes or No

How many different servings of such foods did you have?   _____

If you answered "Yes" to *all* of the questions above (which means you are taking a complete vitamin-mineral supplement *and* also ate at least one serving of the foods listed as being top sources of each of these six important vitamins and minerals), you are probably getting a total of around 150 percent of the RDA for these nutrients. If you are *not* taking a complete vitamin-mineral supplement, you will need to have eaten approximately *four* servings of the foods listed as good sources for each of these nutrients to get at least 100 to 150 percent of the RDA from food. (Please note, some of these foods are sources of *several* of these nutrients—so the one serving of that particular food will count toward all the nutrients for which it is a top source.)

EXERCISE #5   Are You Eating Small Meals throughout the Day and Eating Light at Night?

DIET COMMANDMENT #5
Eat Many Small Meals throughout the Day, and Eat Light at Night

---

With your 1-Day Food Record in front of you, ask yourself these questions:

1. How is my total day's food intake distributed over the day? Do I eat most of my calories in one meal? Two meals? Do I eat most of my food toward the latter part of the day and in the evening?

2. How many meals or snacks did I eat altogether during the day?

3. How big were each of these meals and snacks? Was there a particular time of day when I tended to eat large meals or snacks?

4. What types of food did I eat after 5 P.M., and how much? Would I describe it as a small or a big meal? Would I describe the foods themselves as rich and fried, or light?

EXERCISE #6   Are You Eating at Least Two Calcium-Rich Foods Every Day, Preferably Ones Also High in Vitamin D?

DIET COMMANDMENT #6
Eat at Least Two Calcium-Rich Foods Every Day, Preferably Ones Also High in Vitamin D.

Go back to your 1-Day Food Record and see if any of the foods you ate are listed in Table 10.1. Write the calcium-rich foods that you ate in the spaces below, and write the amount of calcium contributed from each of those foods next to it. Be sure to calculate the amount of calcium for *your* serving size. For example, if you ate 6 ounces of yogurt and the table lists the amount of calcium per 8 ounces (or 1 cup), you need to multiply the amount of calcium in the table by 0.75 (6 ÷ 8) to get the correct amount of calcium for 6 ounces. Similarly, if you ate 3 ounces of cheese and the table lists the amount of calcium for 1 ounce, you need to multiply the amount in the table by 3 to get the correct amount of calcium for your serving.

At the same time that you are noting which calcium-rich foods you ate, check to see if those foods also contain some vitamin D and magnesium as a bonus.

Calcium-Rich Foods You Ate	Calcium (mg)
1. _____	_____
2. _____	_____
3. _____	_____
4. _____	_____
5. _____	_____
6. _____	_____
7. _____	_____
8. _____	_____
9. _____	_____
10. _____	_____
11. _____	_____
12. _____	_____
13. _____	_____
14. _____	_____
15. _____	_____

Now add up the total amount of
calcium you consumed. The total
should be at least 1,200 mg.

Total _____

Table 10.1. Calcium-Rich Foods

Food Source and Serving Size	Calcium (mg)	Fat (g)	Vitamin D (IU)	Magnesium (mg)
Milk and Milk Products				
Buttermilk, 8 oz	284	2.2	5.0	27.0
Chocolate milk, nonfat, 8 oz	292	1.2	100.0	46.0
Chocolate milk, 1% low-fat, 8 oz	288	2.5	100.0	33.0
Chocolate milk, 2% low-fat, 8 oz	285	5.0	100.0	33.0
Chocolate milk, whole, 8 oz	280	8.5	100.0	33.0
Cottage cheese, creamed, small curd, ½ cup	63	4.8	1.0	6.0
Cottage cheese, 2% low-fat, ½ cup	78	2.0	0.5	7.0
Eggnog, 2% low-fat, 8 oz	269	8.0	19.0	32.0
Evaporated milk, nonfat, 4 oz	370	0.3	102.0	34.0
Evaporated milk, 2% low-fat, 4 oz	358	2.5	NA*	33.0
Evaporated milk, whole, canned, 4 oz	329	9.5	100.0	31.0
Half and half cream, 4 oz	127	14.0	20.0	12.0
Lactaid 1% low-fat milk plus calcium, 8 oz	550	2.6	99.0	34.0
Lactose-reduced milk, nonfat, 8 oz	302	0.4	98.0	28.0
Lactose-reduced milk, 1% low-fat, 8 oz	302	2.6	98.0	34.0
Nonfat dry milk powder, with vitamin A added, 1 oz	349	0.2	125.0	33.0
Nonfat milk, with vitamin A added, 8 oz	301	0.4	98.0	28.0
1% low-fat milk, with vitamin A added, 8 oz	300	2.6	98.0	34.0
Sweetened condensed milk, 4 oz	434	13.3	7.0	39.0
2% low-fat milk, with vitamin A added, 8 oz	298	4.7	98.0	33.0
Whole milk, 3.7% fat, 8 oz	290	9.0	98.0	33.0
Yogurt cheese, 1 oz	98	0.8	0.9	8.0
Yogurt, low-fat, custard-style, fruit, 8 oz	373	2.7	3.0	36.0
Yogurt, low-fat, fruit, 8 oz	345	2.5	3.0	33.0
Yogurt, low-fat, plain, 8 oz	415	3.5	4.0	40.0
Yogurt, nonfat, fruit flavor with low-cal sweetener, 8 oz	369	0.4	3.0	41.0

*NA = Not Available

(continued next page)

Table 10.1. (continued)

Food Source and Serving Size	Calcium (mg)	Fat (g)	Vitamin D (IU)	Magnesium (mg)
Yogurt, nonfat, plain, 8 oz	451	0.4	4.0	43.0
Yogurt, nonfat, vanilla or coffee flavor, 8 oz	403	0.4	3.0	39.0
Yogurt, whole milk, plain, 8 oz	274	7.4	4.0	26.0
Other Beverages				
Cocoa mix, Alba sugar-free plus calcium, 1 packet	327	0.5	NA*	43.0
Cocoa mix with dry milk, fortified, 1 packet	100	3.0	NA*	22.0
Hot chocolate/cocoa mix, 1 packet	92	1.0	80.0	24.0
Instant breakfast powder, 1 envelope	106	0.5	2.0	84.0
Sugar-free cocoa mix, unfortified, 1 packet	216	0.5	NA*	31.0
Cheese and Eggs				
American cheese food, 1 oz	141	7.0	8.0	8.4
American cheese, low-fat, 1 oz	194	2.0	0.6	6.8
American processed cheese, 1 oz	175	9.0	2.4	6.3
Brie cheese, 1 oz	52	8.0	2.3	5.7
Cheddar cheese, 1 oz	204	9.4	3.4	7.9
Egg Beaters, ½ cup	63	0.0	0.0	NA*
Feta cheese, 1 oz	140	6.0	5.7	5.4
Monterey jack cheese, 1 oz	211	8.6	2.6	7.6
Mozzarella cheese, part-skim, 1 oz	207	4.8	1.5	7.5
Parmesan cheese, shredded, 1 oz	355	7.7	8.0	14.0
Ricotta cheese, part-skim, 1 oz	77	2.3	0.7	4.2
Scrambled eggs made with milk and margarine, 2	87	15.0	52.0	10.0
Swiss cheese, 1 oz	272	7.8	12.5	10.2
Swiss cheese, low-fat, 1 oz	272	1.5	0.4	10.2
Frozen Desserts				
Banana split, with whipped cream	478	65.0	NA*	89.0
Chocolate-coated ice cream bar, with nuts	136	11.0	2.0	16.0

*NA = Not Available

Table 10.1.   (continued)

Food Source and Serving Size	Calcium (mg)	Fat (g)	Vitamin D (IU)	Magnesium (mg)
Frozen yogurt, low-fat, ½ cup	150	2.0	NA*	38.0
Frozen yogurt, nonfat, chocolate, ½ cup	163	0.0	2.0	39.0
Frozen yogurt, soft-serve, vanilla, ½ cup	103	4.0	1.0	10.0
Fudgsicle ice cream bar	129	0.2	6.0	14.0
Ice cream, premium, vanilla, ½ cup	87	12.0	3.0	8.0
Ice milk, premium, chocolate (Breyer's Light), ½ cup	105	4.0	3.0	14.0
Ice milk, premium, vanilla or strawberry (Breyer's Light), ½ cup	108	4.0	0.3	11.0
Milk shake, all flavors, 8 oz	~260	7.0–8.0	18.0	~30.0
Fish				
Anchovies in oil, drained, 1 oz	66	2.8	11.0	20.0
Bass, freshwater, baked, 3 oz	88	4.0	34.0	32.0
Clams, canned, 3 oz	78	1.7	7.0	15.0
Clams, steamed, 3 oz	78	1.7	7.0	15.0
Crab, steamed, 3 oz	84	5.0	3.0	26.0
Halibut, steamed, 3 oz	51	2.5	34.0	91.0
Herring, baked, 3 oz	90	15.0	105.0	35.0
Herring, smoked, 3 oz	71	10.5	102.0	39.0
Ocean perch, Atlantic, baked, 3 oz	117	1.8	34.0	33.0
Pink salmon, with bones, canned, ½ cup	160	4.5	468.0	26.0
Prawns, breaded and fried, 3 oz	57	10.5	135.0	34.0
Rainbow trout, baked, 3 oz	73	5.0	34.0	26.0
Shrimp, baked, 3 oz	55	4.0	119.0	38.0
Shrimp, canned, 3 oz	50	1.7	146.0	35.0
Fruits				
Dried figs, 3 oz	122	1.0	0.0	50.0

(continued next page)

Table 10.1.   (continued)

Food Source and Serving Size	Nutrient Amounts Provided			
	Calcium (mg)	Fat (g)	Vitamin D (IU)	Magnesium (mg)
Vegetables				
Beet greens, boiled, ½ cup	82	0.1	0.0	49.0
Bok choy, boiled, ½ cup	79	0.1	0.0	9.0
Chinese cabbage, steamed, ½ cup	89	0.2	0.0	16.0
Collard greens, boiled from frozen, ½ cup	179	0.3	0.0	26.0
Dandelion greens, boiled from fresh, ½ cup	74	0.3	0.0	13.0
Rhubarb, fresh, diced, ½ cup	52	0.1	0.0	7.0
Spinach, boiled from frozen, ½ cup	139	0.2	0.0	66.0
Turnip greens, boiled from fresh, ½ cup	99	0.2	0.0	16.0
Vegetarian Breakfast links, 3 oz	54	15.5	0.0	31.0
Veggie Garden burger (meat patty only)	96	3.0	NA*	NA*
Desserts Made with Dairy Products				
Bread pudding with raisins, ½ cup	144	7.0	40.0	24.0
Chocolate mousse, homemade, ½ cup	202	33.0	NA*	44.0
Egg custard, from mix, made with whole milk, ½ cup	194	5.5	0.5	25.0
Pudding, chocolate, instant, made with 2% low-fat milk, ½ cup	153	2.8	NA*	27.0
Pudding, chocolate, instant, made with whole milk, ½ cup	150	4.6	50.0	27.0
Pudding, vanilla, instant, made with 2% low-fat milk, ½ cup	146	2.4	NA*	17.0
Pudding, vanilla, instant, made with whole milk, ½ cup	143	4.0	49.0	17.0
Rice pudding, from mix, made with 2% low-fat milk, ½ cup	151	2.3	NA*	19.0
Rice pudding, from mix, made with whole milk, ½ cup	148	4.0	58.0	19.0
Tapioca pudding, made with 2% low-fat milk, ½ cup	149	2.4	NA*	17.0

*NA = Not Available

Table 10.1.   (continued)

Food Source and Serving Size	Nutrient Amounts Provided			
	Calcium (mg)	Fat (g)	Vitamin D (IU)	Magnesium (mg)
Tapioca pudding, made with whole milk, ½ cup	86	3.6	33.0	11.0
Beans, Peas, and Tofu				
Baked beans, homemade, ½ cup	77	6.5	0.0	54.0
Black-eyed peas, boiled, ½ cup	106	0.3	0.0	43.0
Great northern beans, boiled, ½ cup	60	0.4	0.0	44.0
Navy beans, boiled, ½ cup	64	0.5	0.0	54.0
Red kidney beans, boiled, ½ cup	58	0.1	0.0	42.0
Soybeans, boiled from dry, ½ cup	88	7.7	0.0	74.0
Tofu, firm, ½ cup	258	11.0	0.0	118.0
Tofu, regular, ½ cup	130	6.0	0.0	127.0
White beans, boiled, ½ cup	81	0.3	0.0	57.0
Nuts and Nut Butters				
Almond butter, 2 Tbsp	86	19.0	0.0	97.0
Almonds, toasted, 1 oz	80	14.4	0.0	87.0
Brazilnuts, 1 oz	50	18.8	0.0	64.0
Filberts/hazelnuts, 1 oz	55	19.0	0.0	84.0
Soybeans, dry-roasted, ¼ cup	116	9.3	0.0	98.0
Tahini (sesame butter), 2 Tbsp	128	16.0	0.0	29.0

EXERCISE #7   Is Your Diet Rich in Antioxidants?

> DIET COMMANDMENT #7
> Eat Several Antioxidant-Rich Foods Every Day

Step 1

Go back to your 1-Day Food Record and see if any of the foods you ate are listed in Table 10.2. Write the antioxidant-rich foods that you ate in the spaces below, and write the amount(s) of the three main antioxidants contributed from each of those foods next to it. Be sure to calculate the amount(s) of antioxidants for *your* serving size. For example, if you ate a cup of cantaloupe cubes, and the table lists the amounts of the antioxidants for ½ cup, you simply need to multiply those amounts by 2.

In order to be included here, a food serving has to provide at least 200 RE of beta-carotene (vitamin A), 15 milligrams of vitamin C, *or* 2 milligrams of vitamin E. If a food you ate is *not* listed in this table, it probably doesn't provide enough of these nutrients to qualify as antioxidant-rich (though it may provide some).

Antioxidant-Rich Foods You Ate	Beta-Carotene (vitamin A) (RE)	Vitamin C (mg)	Vitamin E (mg)
1.			
2.			
3.			
4.			
5.			
6.			
7.			
8.			
9.			
10.			
	Total	Total	Total

Step 2

Now add up the total amounts you consumed of each of these three main antioxidants. Then compare your consumption against the RDAs. And ask yourself these questions:

- Am I eating several antioxidant-rich foods every day?
- Am I getting at least 100 percent of the RDA for each of them?
- Am I getting two to three times the RDA?

The RDA for vitamin A in total (which includes beta-carotene) is 800 RE; for vitamin C, 60 milligrams; and for vitamin E, 8 milligrams (12 IU).

Table 10.2. Antioxidant-Rich Foods

Food Source and Serving Size	Beta-Carotene (Vitamin A) (RE)	Vitamin C (mg)	Vitamin E (mg)
Fruits			
Apricot halves, ½ cup	202		
Apricots, dried halves, ¼ cup	235		2.0
Blackberries, ½ cup		15	
Blueberries, frozen, 1 cup			3.0
Boysenberries, fresh, ½ cup		15	
Breadfruit, ½ cup		32	
Cantaloupe/muskmelon, cubed, ½ cup	258	34	
Carambola/star fruit		27	
Elderberries, fresh, ½ cup		26	
Grapefruit, pink/red, half		47	
Grapefruit sections, canned in juice, ½ cup		42	
Grapefruit, white, half		39	
Guava, half		83	
Honeydew melon, cubed, ½ cup		21	
Kiwi		57	
Lemon, peeled		31	
Loganberries, fresh, ½ cup		16	
Mango	805	57	2.0
Mango slices, ½ cup	642	46	2.0
Orange, California		80	
Orange, Florida		68	
Orange, medium		70	
Orange sections, ½ cup		48	
Papaya, half		94	
Papaya slices, ½ cup		43	
Prunes, dried, 10			2.0
Red raspberries, ½ cup		15	
Strawberries, sliced, ½ cup		47	
Strawberries, whole, ½ cup		41	
Tangelo, medium		51	

(*continued next page*)

Table 10.2. (continued)

Food Source and Serving Size	Beta-Carotene (Vitamin A) (RE)	Vitamin C (mg)	Vitamin E (mg)
Tangerine		26	
Tangerine sections, ½ cup		30	
Fruit and Vegetable Juices			
Apple juice, with vitamin C, 8 oz		103	
Cranberry-apricot drink, low-cal, 8 oz		77	
Cranberry-apricot drink, with vitamin C, 8 oz		81	
Cranberry juice cocktail, 8 oz		90	
Cranberry juice cocktail, low-cal, 8 oz		77	
Grapefruit juice, canned, 8 oz		72	
Grapefruit juice, fresh, 8 oz		94	
Grapefruit juice, from concentrate, 8 oz		83	
Orange juice, fresh, 8 oz		124	
Orange juice, from concentrate, 8 oz		97	
Pineapple juice, from concentrate, 10 oz		38	
Pineapple juice, with vitamin C, canned, 8 oz		96	
Strawberry juice, 8 oz		67	
Tangerine juice, fresh, 8 oz		77	
Tangerine juice, from concentrate, 8 oz		77	
Vegetable juice cocktail (V-8), 8 oz		67	
Vegetable juice cocktail (V-8), low-sodium, 8 oz		67	
Yellow passion fruit juice, 8 oz	588		
Vegetables			
Asparagus, boiled from frozen, ½ cup		22	
Asparagus, cooked from fresh, ½ cup		24	25
Bell pepper, green, half	23	27	
Bell pepper, sweet red, raw, half	211	70	
Bell pepper, yellow, half	22	171	
Bell peppers, sweet red, chopped, ½ cup	285	95	
Bok choy, boiled, ½ cup	219	22	
Broccoflower, steamed, ½ cup		49	
Broccoli florets, raw, 3 oz	255	79	

Table 10.2.   (continued)

Food Source and Serving Size	Beta-Carotene (Vitamin A) (RE)	Vitamin C (mg)	Vitamin E (mg)
Broccoli pieces, cooked, 1 cup	216	116	2.0
Broccoli pieces, raw, ½ cup		41	
Brussels sprouts, boiled, ½ cup		48	
Cabbage, chopped and steamed, ½ cup		21	
Cabbage, kimchee-style, ½ cup	240		
Cabbage, red, boiled, ½ cup		26	
Carrot	2,024		
Carrot slices, steamed, ½ cup	1,977		
Carrots, raw, grated, ¼ cup	774		
Cauliflower, boiled, ½ cup		34	
Cauliflower, raw, ½ cup		36	
Chili peppers, hot red, canned, ¼ cup	404	23	
Chili pepper, hot red, raw, ¼ cup	403	91	
Chinese cabbage, steamed, ½ cup	242	33	
Dried mixed vegetables (Salad Crunchies), 2 Tbsp	392	28	
Green peas, edible pods, cooked from fresh, 1 cup		77	5.0
Greens			
Beet, boiled, 1 cup	734	36	2.0
Chicory, raw, chopped, 1 cup	720	22	NA*
Dandelion, boiled, 1 cup	1,228	19	2.0
Dandelion, raw, 1 cup	770	19	
Dock/sorrel, cooked, 1 cup	347	26	NA*
Dock/sorrel, raw, chopped, 1 cup	532	64	NA*
Mustard, boiled from frozen, 1 cup	670	36	3.0
Turnip, boiled, 1 cup	792	40	2.5
Jicama, raw, ½ cup			3.0
Jute/potherb, boiled, ½ cup	223		
Kale, boiled, ½ cup	481	27	3.7
Kale, raw, chopped, ½ cup	298	40	2.7

*NA = Not Available

(continued next page)

Table 10.2. (continued)

Food Source and Serving Size	Beta-Carotene (Vitamin A) (RE)	Vitamin C (mg)	Vitamin E (mg)
Kohlrabi, boiled, ½ cup		45	
Lamb's-quarters, boiled, ½ cup	872		
Lamb's-quarters, raw, chopped, ½ cup	324		
Lettuce, romaine, 3 oz	221		
Peas and carrots, boiled from frozen, ½ cup	621		
Peas, raw, ½ cup		29	1.0
Pumpkin, fresh, boiled, ½ cup	1,326		1.0
Pumpkin/squash mix, canned, ½ cup	2,710		
Radish, white icicle, raw slices, ½ cup		15	
Rutabaga, raw cubes, ½ cup		18	
Salsa/Mexican sauce, homemade, ½ cup		43	
Seaweed (laver/nori), ½ cup	208		
Snow peas, steamed, ½ cup		42	
Spinach, boiled, ½ cup	737	9	2.0
Spinach, fresh, chopped, 2 cups	752	32	3.0
Squash			
Acorn, baked cubes, 1 cup		22	
Butternut, baked and mashed, ½ cup	858	19	
Butternut, baked cubes, 1 cup	1,435	31	
Hubbard, baked cubes, 1 cup	1,449	23	
Hubbard, boiled and mashed, ½ cup	473		
Succotash, cooked, 1 cup			2.0
Sweet potato, baked, without skin	2,574	26	6.0
Sweet potato, canned, ½ cup	1,936		4.5
Swiss chard, boiled, 1 cup	550	32	3.0
Tomatoes, fresh, chopped, ½ cup		17	
Winter squash, baked and mashed, ½ cup	545	14	
Winter squash, baked cubes, 1 cup	730	20	
Yams, orange, mashed, ½ cup	2,182	25	
Beans and Bean Products			
Garbanzo beans, cooked from dry, 1 cup			2.0
Lima beans, canned, 1 cup			3.0

Table 10.2. (continued)

Food Source and Serving Size	Beta-Carotene (Vitamin A) (RE)	Vitamin C (mg)	Vitamin E (mg)
Lima beans, cooked from dry, 1 cup			6.0
Lima beans, cooked from frozen, 1 cup			3.0
Navy beans, cooked from dry, 1 cup			2.0
Soybeans, cooked from dry, 1 cup			12.0
Tofu, ½ cup			4.0
White beans, cooked from dry, 1 cup			2.0
*Breads and Cereal Products**			
Carrot muffin, with raisins, 3 oz	356		
Cold Cereals			
All Bran, ½ cup	570	23	
Bran Chex, 1 cup		26	
Corn Flakes, 1 cup	300	12	
Cracklin' Oat Bran, 1 cup	454	32	
Fiber One, 1 cup		30	
Nutri-Grain Corn, 1 cup	556	22	11.0
Nutri-Grain Wheat, 1 cup	583	23	12.0
100% Bran cereal, ½ cup		31	
Product 19, 1 cup	1,747	70	35.0
Total Corn Flakes, 1 cup	1,747	70	35.0
Total Wheat cereal, 1 cup	1,747	70	35.0
Wheat Chex, 1 cup		24	
Cornbread muffin			2.0
Wheat germ, toasted, 2 Tbsp			2.8
Eggs			
Egg substitute, ½ cup	258		
Fish, Entrees, and Fried Foods			
Burrito, any type			2.0
Catfish, breaded and baked, 3 oz			2.0
Chicken chow mein, 1 cup			8.0
Chicken enchilada, low-cal frozen meal		92	

*Many cereal brands are fortified with vitamin A/beta-carotene, vitamin C, and vitamin E; check the labels on your favorite cereals.

(continued next page)

Table 10.2. (continued)

Food Source and Serving Size	Beta-Carotene (Vitamin A) (RE)	Vitamin C (mg)	Vitamin E (mg)
Chicken pot pie, cooked from frozen			4.0
Chili relleño	641	89	2.0
Clam sauce, ½ cup			3.0
Clams, canned, drained, ½ cup		18	
Clams, steamed, 3 oz		19	
Enchilada, any type			2.0
Fish sandwich (fast-food)			2.0
Macaroni and cheese, homemade, 1 cup			3.5
Manicotti, cooked from frozen			2.0
Ocean perch, breaded and fried, 3 oz			2.0
Quiche lorraine, ⅛ of 9" pie			5.5
Salmon, sockeye, broiled, 3 oz			2.0
Scallops, breaded and fried, 3 oz			2.0
Sea bass, baked and broiled, 3 oz			2.0
Shrimp/prawns, breaded and fried, 3 oz			3.0
Shrimp salad, ½ cup			4.0
Spaghetti, with marinara sauce, 1 cup			5.0
Turkey pot pie, cooked from frozen			3.0
Vegetable lasagna, frozen meal		62	
Soups and Stews			
Beef and vegetable stew, homemade, 1 cup			2.0
Chicken vegetable soup, 1 cup	602		
Chunky chicken rice soup, ½ can	656		
Chunky vegetable soup, 1 cup	288		
Tomato soup, with milk or water, 8 oz		62	
Nuts and Seeds			
Almond butter, 2 Tbsp			6.0
Almonds, oil-roasted, 1 oz			8.0
Filberts/hazelnuts, dry-roasted, 1 oz			7.0
Peanut butter and jelly sandwich			2.5
Peanut butter, smooth or chunky, 2 Tbsp			2.0
Peanuts, dry-roasted, 1 oz			2.0

Table 10.2. (continued)

Food Source and Serving Size	Beta-Carotene (Vitamin A) (RE)	Vitamin C (mg)	Vitamin E (mg)
Soybeans, roasted, ½ cup			5.0
Sunflower seed butter, 2 Tbsp			15.0
Sunflower seed kernels, roasted, 2 Tbsp			10.0
Oils			
Almond oil, 1 Tbsp			5.0
Canola oil, 1 Tbsp			3.0
Corn oil, 1 Tbsp			3.0
Cottonseed oil, 1 Tbsp			5.0
Hazelnut oil, 1 Tbsp			6.0
Olive oil, 1 Tbsp			2.0
Peanut oil, 1 Tbsp			2.0
Rice bran oil, 1 Tbsp			5.0
Safflower oil, 1 Tbsp			5.0
Soybean oil, 1 Tbsp			2.0
Sunflower oil, 1 Tbsp			8.0
Items Made with Oil			
Cake, chocolate, 3 oz			2.5
Cake, white, 3 oz			2.5
Cake, yellow, 3 oz			2.5
Carrot cake, with frosting, 1 piece			6.0
Cinnamon coffee cake, with crumb topping, 3 oz			2.5
Corn fritter, homemade			3.5
Pesto sauce, ¼ cup			3.0
Salad Dressings			
French, 1 Tbsp			4.0
Italian, 1 Tbsp			4.0
Ranch, 1 Tbsp			2.5
Russian, 1 Tbsp			4.0
1,000 Island, 1 Tbsp			5.0
Vinegar and oil, 1 Tbsp			3.0

(*continued next page*)

Table 10.2. (continued)

Food Source and Serving Size	Beta-Carotene (Vitamin A) (RE)	Vitamin C (mg)	Vitamin E (mg)
Margarines			
Fleischmann's, from tub, 1 Tbsp			2.0
Imperial, from tub, 1 Tbsp			2.0
Parkay Soft, from tub, 1 Tbsp			2.0
Promise, Extra Light, 1 Tbsp			3.0
Promise, spread, 1 Tbsp			3.0
Saffola, from stick, 1 Tbsp			3.0
Saffola, from tub, 1 Tbsp			2.0
Mayonnaise Products			
Mayonnaise, 1 Tbsp			4.0
Mayonnaise (Saffola), 1 Tbsp			3.0
Tartar sauce, 1 Tbsp			2.0
Items Made with Mayonnaise			
Avocado and cheese sandwich			5.0
Bacon, lettuce, and tomato sandwich			4.0
Carrot-raisin salad, ½ cup			5.0
Chicken salad sandwich			8.0
Coleslaw, ½ cup			2.0
Egg salad, ½ cup			8.0
Egg salad sandwich			8.0
Ham salad sandwich			5.0
Ham sandwich on white			3.5
Macaroni salad, ½ cup			6.0
Roast beef sandwich			3.0
Tuna salad sandwich			4.5
Turkey sandwich on whole-wheat			3.0
Waldorf salad, ½ cup			5.0

EXERCISE #8   Are You Eating Too Much Fat?

DIET COMMANDMENT #8
Eat No More Than 20 to 25 Percent of Your Calories from Fat

Step 1

Using Table A.6 in appendix A, write down the calories and the fat, protein, and sodium content of every food you listed in your 1-Day Food Record, which includes columns for all these categories of information. (We'll get to sodium in Exercise #10, but save yourself some time later by writing it down now.) Remember to calculate the amount of calories and the fat, protein, and sodium contents for *your* particular serving of each food.

- If you ate a supermarket product that isn't listed in Table A.6, write down the amounts of calories, fat, protein, and sodium listed on its product label. As of May 1994, most supermarket products are required by the Food and Drug Administration (FDA) to list this information on the package label.
- If you ate a dish that isn't listed in this table, do your best to find the closest match, or look up separately the individual foods that make up the dish. For example, if you ate some creamy curry chicken, you could look up the amount of rice, then chicken, and then cream sauce. In the case of mushu pork (a popular dish in Chinese restaurants), you could look up a flour tortilla for the Chinese crepe, and then look up pork, mixed vegetables, and scrambled egg.

Once you have looked up and written down this information for every food you ate, total up the amounts of calories, fat, and protein you consumed.

Step 2: Calculating the Percent of Your Calories from Fat

Write down in the appropriate space below the total grams of fat you consumed during the day. Multiply this number by 9 (because there are 9 calories per gram of fat), and write the result below. Take this new number, and divide it by the total number of calories you consumed during the same day. Multiply by 100 (or simply move the decimal point two places to the right) to get your "percent of calories from fat."

_____ × 9 = _____

Total grams of fat consumed	Total calories from fat

_____ ÷ _____ = _____

Total calories from fat	Total number of calories consumed	Portion of calories from fat

_____ × 100 = _____%

Portion of calories from fat	Percent of calories from fat

Table 10.3. High-Fiber Foods

Food Source and Serving Size	Fiber (g)
Fruits	
Apple rings, dried, 1.5 oz	3.7
Apple with peel, large	5.7
Apple with peel, medium	3.7
Apricots, 2	1.6
Apricots, dried halves, 1.5 oz	3.8
Apricots, dried halves, cooked, ½ cup	4.2
Banana	2.7
Banana chips, ½ cup	3.5
Banana slices, ½ cup	1.8
Blackberries/boysenberries, fresh or frozen, ½ cup	3.5
Blueberries, frozen, ½ cup	2.4
Chayote	6.1
Cherries, ½ cup	1.2
Cranberries, ½ cup	2.0
Currants, dried (Zante), ½ cup	4.9
Dates, chopped, ½ cup	6.7
Dates, whole, 1.5 oz	3.2
Elderberries, cooked and canned, ½ cup	6.6
Figs, cooked from dried, ½ cup	6.2
Figs, fresh, 3	5.0
Fruit salad, with no citrus fruits, ½ cup	1.5
Gooseberries, canned, ½ cup	3.0
Grapefruit, pink/red, half	1.6
Grapes, 1 cup	1.0
Kiwifruit	2.6
Loganberries, frozen or fresh, ½ cup	3.6
Melon	
Cantaloupe/muskmelon, cubed, 1 cup	1.2
Casaba/crenshaw melon, cubed, 1 cup	1.4
Honeydew melon, cubed, 1 cup	1.0
Mixed fruit, dried, 1.5 oz	1.8
Orange, large	4.4
Orange, medium	3.2
Papaya, fresh	5.5
Peach, medium	1.8

Table 10.3. (continued)

Food Source and Serving Size	Fiber (g)
Peaches, dried halves, 1.5 oz	3.5
Pear, bosc, small	3.3
Pear, D'Anjou, large	5.0
Pears, Asian or Bartlett	4.0
Pears, dried halves, 1.5 oz	2.0
Pears in juice, canned, ½ cup	2.5
Pear slices, ½ cup	2.0
Persimmon, Japanese, large	6.1
Pineapple, in juice, ½ cup	0.9
Plum, medium	1.0
Plum slices, ½ cup	1.2
Pomegranate	1.0
Prunes, dried, 1.5 oz	3.0
Raisins, ¼ cup	1.7
Red raspberries, ½ cup	2.8
Strawberries, fresh, ½ cup	1.9
Strawberries, frozen, ½ cup	2.4
Tangelo, medium	2.3
Tomatillo, chopped, ½ cup	1.3
Tomato, stewed, ½ cup	2.0
Tomato, sun-dried, 5 pieces	1.2
Vegetables	
Artichoke globe, boiled	6.5
Artichoke hearts, fresh, ½ cup	5.0
Asparagus pieces, cooked, ½ cup	1.9
Avocado cubes, ½ cup	4.4
Bamboo shoots, sliced, raw, ½ cup	1.7
Bean sprouts, mung, cooked, ½ cup	2.1
Bean sprouts, mung, raw, ½ cup	1.0
Beets, canned, ½ cup	1.5
Broccoli pieces, boiled, ½ cup	2.7
Brussels sprouts, cooked, ½ cup	3.4
Cabbage, savoy, cooked, ½ cup	1.7
Cabbage, savoy, raw, ½ cup	1.1

(*continued next page*)

Table 10.3. (continued)

Food Source and Serving Size	Fiber (g)
Carrot, raw	2.2
Carrots, cooked, ½ cup	2.6
Cauliflower, boiled, ½ cup	2.0
Cauliflower, raw, ½ cup	1.3
Celery root, boiled, ½ cup	3.0
Chili pepper, hot green, canned	1.4
Corn on the cob, cooked	2.1
Corn, white, cooked from frozen, ½ cup	2.5
Corn, yellow, canned, ½ cup	6.0
Corn, yellow, cooked, ½ cup	2.3
Cucumber, medium	0.7
Eggplant, cubed, cooked, ½ cup	1.2
Green beans, boiled from fresh, ½ cup	2.0
Green beans, Italian, cooked from frozen, ½ cup	2.2
Green peas, canned, ½ cup	3.5
Green peas, cooked from frozen, ½ cup	4.4
Greens	
Beet, boiled, ½ cup	2.0
Beet/collard, raw, ½ cup	0.7
Chicory, raw, chopped, ½ cup	3.4
Collard, boiled, ½ cup	1.3
Collard, cooked from frozen, ½ cup	2.9
Dandelion, boiled, ½ cup	1.5
Dock/sorrel, raw, chopped, ½ cup	1.9
Mustard, boiled, ½ cup	1.5
Turnip, cooked from frozen, ½ cup	3.5
Jalapeño peppers, chopped, canned, ¼ cup	1.0
Jicama, fresh slices, ½ cup	2.1
Kale, boiled, ½ cup	1.3
Kale, fresh, chopped, ½ cup	1.0
Kohlrabi, boiled, ½ cup	1.0
Kohlrabi slices, fresh, ½ cup	2.5
Leeks, chopped, cooked, ½ cup	1.7
Lettuce	
Butterhead or iceberg, chopped, 2 cups	1.5
Green leaf, chopped, 2 cups	1.6

Table 10.3. (continued)

Food Source and Serving Size	Fiber (g)
Romaine, chopped, 2 cups	2.0
Spinach, chopped, 2 cups	3.8
Mixed vegetables, cooked from frozen, ½ cup	4.9
Mushrooms, boiled, ½ cup	1.7
Mushrooms, shiitake, cooked, ½ cup	1.5
Okra pods, cooked from frozen, ½ cup	2.6
Parsnips, fresh or boiled, ½ cup	3.3
Pepper, red or green bell, chopped, ½ cup	1.0
Pepper, yellow, large	4.3
Potato, large, with skin	4.4
Potato, medium, peeled after boiling	2.4
Potato, medium, with skin	2.9
Rhubarb, cooked, ½ cup	2.4
Rutabaga cubes, fresh, ½ cup	1.8
Sauerkraut, canned, ½ cup	3.0
Snow peas, cooked from frozen, ½ cup	2.6
Spinach, canned, drained, ½ cup	2.9
Spinach, cooked from frozen, ½ cup	2.9
Squash	
Acorn squash, baked, mashed, ½ cup	5.3
Acorn squash, cooked cubes, ½ cup	4.5
Hubbard squash, mashed, ½ cup	3.4
Succotash, boiled from fresh, ½ cup	4.9
Summer squash slices, raw, ½ cup	1.2
Sweet potatoes, candied, ½ cup	1.9
Sweet potatoes, canned, mashed, ½ cup	3.8
Sweet potato, medium, cooked and peeled	3.6
Swiss chard, boiled, ½ cup	1.8
Turnip cubes, boiled, ½ cup	1.6
Turnip cubes, fresh, ½ cup	1.2
Water chestnuts, ½ cup	1.8
Yams, orange, mashed, ½ cup	3.0
Yams, white, cooked cubes, ½ cup	2.7
Yellow wax beans, canned, ½ cup	0.9
Yellow wax beans, cooked from frozen, ½ cup	2.1

(*continued next page*)

Table 10.3. (continued)

Food Source and Serving Size	Fiber (g)
Fruit and Vegetable Juices	
Apricot nectar, 8 oz	1.0
Carrot juice, canned, 8 oz	2.0
Grapefruit juice, bottled, 8 oz	0.7
Low-sodium tomato juice, 8 oz	2.0
Orange juice, fresh, 8 oz	1.0
Orange juice, from concentrate, 8 oz	0.5
Peach, pear, or papaya nectar, 8 oz	1.5
Pineapple juice, bottled, 8 oz	0.7
Vegetable juice cocktail (V-8), 8 oz	1.9
Beans and Bean Products	
Baby lima beans, cooked from frozen, ½ cup	6.0
Black beans, cooked, ½ cup	7.7
Black-eyed peas, boiled from fresh, ½ cup	4.1
Chili with beans, canned, ½ cup	4.1
Great northern beans, cooked, ½ cup	5.4
Kidney beans, red, cooked, ½ cup	7.5
Lima beans, canned, drained, ½ cup	5.4
Navy beans, cooked, ½ cup	8.0
Pinto beans, cooked, ½ cup	9.8
Pork and beans, canned with tomato sauce, ½ cup	7.0
Refried beans, canned, ½ cup	11.0
Soybeans, cooked, ½ cup	3.0
White beans, cooked, ½ cup	7.0
Yard-long beans, cooked, ½ cup	1.4
Bread Products	
Blueberry muffin	1.6
Bran muffin	2.8
English muffin, plain or sourdough	1.5
French or Italian bread, per slice	1.0
Hamburger or hot dog bun	1.2
Mixed-grain bread (not with whole-wheat flour as the first ingredient), per slice	1.8
Pita pocket bread, white	1.0
Pita pocket bread, whole-wheat	3.4
Pumpernickel bread, per slice	1.9

Table 10.3. (continued)

Food Source and Serving Size	Fiber (g)
Sourdough bread, per slice	0.7
Submarine (Hoagie) roll	2.2
Rye bread, per slice	1.6
White bread, per slice	0.5
Wheat, cracked-wheat, or wheat-berry bread, per slice	1.2
Whole-wheat bread, per slice	2.4
Whole-wheat roll	2.5
Cold Cereals	
All Bran, ½ cup	10.0
All Bran Extra Fiber, ½ cup	15.0
Almond Delight, 1 cup	4.0
Apple Jacks, 1 cup	1.0
Banana Nut Crunch, 1 cup	4.0
Basic 4, 1 cup	3.0
Blueberry Morning, 1¼ cups	2.0
Blueberry Muesli, 1 cup	4.0
Bran Buds, ½ cup	11.7
Cap 'n Crunch (assorted types), ¾ cup	1.0
Cheerios, 1 cup	3.0
Cheerios, Apple Cinnamon, ¾ cup	1.0
Cheerios, Honey Nut, 1 cup	2.0
Cheerios, Multi Grain, 1 cup	3.0
Cinnamon Toast Crunch, ¾ cup	1.0
Clusters, 1 cup	4.0
Complete Bran Flakes, ¾ cup	5.0
Corn Flakes, Kellogg's, 1 cup	1.0
Corn Pops, 1 cup	1.0
Cracklin Oat Bran, ¾ cup	6.0
Crispix, 1 cup	1.0
Crunchy Corn Bran, ¾ cup	5.0
CW Post, 1 cup	3.0
Fiber One, ½ cup	13.0
Frosted Mini-Wheats, 1 cup	6.0
Frosted Mini-Wheats, Bite Size, 1 cup	6.0
Frosted Wheat Bites, 1 cup	5.0

(*continued next page*)

Table 10.3. (continued)

Food Source and Serving Size	Fiber (g)
Fruit & Fibre, Dates & Walnuts, 1 cup	6.0
Fruit & Fibre, Peaches & Almonds, 1 cup	6.0
Fruitful Bran, 1 cup	6.7
Fruit Loops, 1 cup	1.0
Golden Grahams, ¾ cup	1.0
Grapenut Flakes, ¾ cup	3.0
Grapenuts, ½ cup	5.0
Great Grains Crunchy Pecan, ⅔ cup	4.0
Great Grains Raisin, Date & Pecan, ⅔ cup	4.0
Healthy Choice Multi Grain Flakes, 1 cup	3.0
Healthy Choice Multi Grain Squares, 1¼ cups	6.0
Healthy Choice Raisin & Crunchy Clusters, 1¼ cups	4.0
Honey Bunches of Oats, ¾ cup	1.0
Honey Comb, 1⅓ cups	1.0
Honey Graham Oh's, ¾ cup	1.0
Just Right Crunchy Nugget, 1 cup	3.0
Just Right Fruit and Nut, 1 cup	3.0
Kashi Medley, ½ cup	2.0
Kashi, Puffed, 1 cup	2.0
Kellogg's Lowfat Granola, ½ cup	3.0
Kellogg's Lowfat Granola with Raisins, ⅔ cup	3.0
Kix, 1⅓ cups	1.0
Kix, Berry Berry, ¾ cup	1.0
Life, Cinnamon, 1 cup	4.0
Life, Oat, ¾ cup	2.0
Lucky Charms, 1 cup	1.0
Natural Bran Flakes, ⅔ cup	6.0
Nature Valley Granola, 1 cup	12.0
Mueslix Golden Crunch, ⅔ cup	6.0
Mueslix Raisin & Date, ⅔ cup	4.0
Multi Bran Chex, 1¼ cups	7.0
Nutri-Grain Almond Raisin, 1¼ cups	4.0
Nutri-Grain Golden Wheat, ¾ cup	4.0
Nutri-Grain Golden Wheat with Raisins, 1¼ cups	6.0
Oatmeal Crisp Apple Cinnamon, 1 cup	3.0
Oatmeal Crisp with Almonds, 1 cup	3.0
Oatmeal Crisp with Raisins, 1 cup	2.0

Table 10.3. (continued)

Food Source and Serving Size	Fiber (g)
Oat Squares, 1 cup	4.0
100% Bran, 1/3 cup	8.0
100% Natural Oats, Honey & Raisins (Crist Mill), 1/2 cup	4.0
Puffed Wheat, 1 cup	2.3
Quaker 100% Natural, Low Fat, 1/2 cup	3.0
Quaker 100% Natural Oats & Honey, 1/2 cup	4.0
Quaker 100% Natural Oats, Honey, Raisins, 1/2 cup	4.0
Raisin Bran, Kellogg's, 1 cup	7.0
Raisin Bran, Post, 1 cup	8.0
Raisin Nut Bran, 1 cup	5.0
Raisin Squares, 3/4 cup	5.0
Rice Krispies, 1 1/4 cups	1.0
Rice Krispies Apple Cinnamon, 3/4 cup	1.0
Shredded Wheat, 2 biscuits	5.0
Shredded Wheat 'n Bran, 1 1/4 cups	8.0
Shredded Wheat Spoonsize, 1 cup	5.0
Shredded Wheat (Sunshine), 2 biscuits	6.0
Smacks, 3/4 cup	1.0
Special K, 1 cup	1.0
Sun Crunchers, 1 cup	3.0
Toasted Oatmeal, 2/3 cup	2.0
Toasted Oatmeal, Honey Nut, 1 cup	3.0
Total Raisin Bran, 1 cup	5.0
Total Whole Grain, 3/4 cup	3.0
Wheaties, 1 cup	3.0
Wheaties Honey Gold, 3/4 cup	1.0
Wheat Chex, whole grain, 3/4 cup	5.0
Wheat Total with Calcium, 1 cup	2.4
Hot Cereal	
Corn grits, 1 cup	4.5
Cream of rice, 1 cup	1.4
Cream of wheat, 1 cup	3.4
Farina, 1 cup	3.2
Malt-O-Meal, 1 cup	3.0
Maypo, 3/4 cup	2.2

(*continued next page*)

Table 10.3. (continued)

Food Source and Serving Size	Fiber (g)
Millet, cooked, ½ cup	1.3
Oatmeal, homemade, 1 cup	4.1
Oatmeal, instant, fortified, ¾ cup	3.0
Ralston cereal, 1 cup	3.3
Roman Meal, ¾ cup	5.6
Wheatena, 1 cup	3.3
Whole-wheat cereal, 1 cup	3.9
Grain Products	
Barley, cooked, 1 cup	4.5
Bulgur wheat, cooked, 1 cup	10.6
Cornbread, 1 serving	2.3
Crackers	
Armenian cracker bread, 4	3.7
Rye, whole-grain crackers, 4	4.4
Whole-wheat crackers, 4	1.6
Noodles	
Corn-based noodles, cooked, ½ cup	2.9
Noodles, enriched, cooked, ½ cup	1.0
Whole-wheat noodles, cooked, ½ cup	3.1
Oat bran, ½ cup	8.2
Pancakes, buckwheat, 3	3.9
Pancakes, plain or buttermilk, 3	1.2
Pancakes, whole-wheat, 3	7.2
Popcorn, popped, plain, 1 cup	1.3
Pretzels, thin twists, 10	1.7
Rice	
Brown rice, cooked, ½ cup	1.8
Rice and pasta (Rice A Roni), cooked, ½ cup	4.3
Spanish rice, ½ cup	1.6
White rice, cooked, ½ cup	0.5
White rice, glutinous, sticky, cooked, ½ cup	1.2
Rice bran, 1 oz	21.7
Stove Top Stuffing, ½ cup	3.1
Tortilla, corn, 6″ diameter	2.4
Tortilla, flour, 8″ diameter	1.0
Waffles, frozen, 4″ diameter, 2	1.6

Table 10.3. (continued)

Food Source and Serving Size	Fiber (g)
Waffles, 7" diameter	1.1
Wheat bran, ½ cup	7.6
Fruit Desserts	
Fruit crisp, 3" x 3"	2.0
Fruit pie, ⅙ of 9" pie	~2.5
Pumpkin pie, 1 piece	5.4
Nuts and Seeds	
Almond butter, 2 Tbsp	1.2
Almonds, toasted, 1 oz	3.2
Cashews, dry-roasted, 4 Tbsp	1.0
Coconut, dried, ½ cup	6.5
Coconut, freshly grated, ½ cup	3.6
Coconut, shredded, sweetened, packaged, 1.5 oz	1.9
Macadamia nuts, roasted, 4 Tbsp	3.1
Mixed nuts, dry-roasted, 4 Tbsp	3.1
Peanut butter, chunky, 2 Tbsp	2.1
Peanut butter, smooth, 2 Tbsp	1.9
Peanuts, dry-roasted, 4 Tbsp	3.0
Pecans, dry-roasted, 4 Tbsp	2.4
Pumpkin kernels, roasted, 4 Tbsp	5.9
Sunflower seed butter, 2 Tbsp	4.1
Sunflower seeds, dry-roasted, 4 Tbsp	2.9
Tahini (sesame butter), 2 Tbsp	2.8
Walnut halves, dried, 4 Tbsp	1.2
Other Vegetable Products and Dishes	
Coleslaw, 1 cup	2.4
French fries, from frozen, ½ cup	0.9
Hash brown potatoes, cooked, ½ cup	1.6
Mashed potatoes, ½ cup	2.4
Potato chips, 1 oz	1.5
Potatoes au gratin, ½ cup	2.2
Potato salad, 1 cup	3.7
Tater tots, ½ cup	2.0
Waldorf salad, 1 cup	3.6

(*continued next page*)

Table 10.3. (continued)

Food Source and Serving Size	Fiber (g)
Soups and Stews	
Bean and bacon soup, 1 cup	2.6
Beef and vegetable stew, homemade, 1 cup	3.4
Black bean soup, 1 cup	2.0
Chicken noodle soup, 1 cup	0.7
Clam chowder, 1 cup	1.0
Green pea soup, 1 cup	1.2
Lentil and ham soup, 1 cup	1.9
Minestrone soup, 1 cup	1.0
Potato soup, 1 cup	0.9
Split pea soup, chunky, 1 cup	1.6
Tomato rice soup, 1 cup	0.8
Turkey soup, 1 cup	1.0
Vegetable beef soup, 1 cup	0.8
Vegetarian vegetable soup, 1 cup	1.6
Mixed Dishes	
Bean burrito	8.2
Beef and bean burrito	5.0
Chicken chow mein, homemade, 1 cup	4.1
Enchilada	2.0
Lasagna, 1 serving	1.6
Macaroni and cheese, 1 cup	1.3
Macaroni salad, 1 cup	1.3
Moussaka (lamb and eggplant), 1 cup	5.6
Pizza, regular-crust, per slice	2.2
Pizza, thick-crust, per slice	4.2
Spaghetti, with marinara sauce, 1 cup	2.5
Stuffed cabbage rolls, 8 oz	3.5
Stuffed green pepper	1.4
Taco	1.1
Tostada with beans	6.9
Tostada with beans and beef	4.0
Tostada with beans and chicken	3.7

Question to ask yourself:

Are you getting 20 percent or less of your calories from fat?

Step 3: Calculating the Percent of Your Calories from Protein

Write down in the appropriate space below the total grams of protein you consumed during the day. Multiply this number by 4 (because there are 4 calories per gram of protein), and write the result below. Take this new number, and divide it by the total number of calories you consumed during the same day. Multiply by 100 (or simply move the decimal point two places to the right) to get your "percent of calories from protein."

_____ × 4 = _____

Total grams of protein consumed	Total calories from protein

_____ ÷ _____ = _____

Total calories from protein	Total number of calories consumed	Portion of calories from protein

_____ × 100 = _____%

Portion of calories from protein	Percent of calories from protein

Question to ask yourself:

Are you getting around 15 percent of your calories from protein?

EXERCISE #9   Are You Eating Enough Fiber?

DIET COMMANDMENT #9
Eat 20 to 30 Grams of Fiber Every Day, from a Variety of Different Foods

Step 1

Go through Table 10.3, looking up all the foods listed in your 1-Day Food Record. Write down the amount of fiber for each food listed, based on your particular serving size. Only foods containing *1 gram of fiber or more* per typical serving are included in Table 10.3. If a particular food or product is *not* listed in this table, write down the amount of fiber listed on its nutrition information label, if available, or write down the amount of fiber listed for a similar food.

Step 2

Add up the total grams of fiber you consumed during the day. Did you consume 20 to 30 grams of fiber, thus satisfying Diet Commandment #9?

EXERCISE #10   Are You Moderating Your Intake of Sodium and Sugar?

> DIET COMMANDMENT #10
> Moderate Your Intake of Sodium and Sugar

In Exercise #8, you went through Table A.6 in appendix A and wrote down the amounts of fat and protein you consumed. Now you're going to do the same thing for sodium, then look at a new table for sugar.

Step 1

Referring again to Table A.6, write down the sodium content of each of the foods listed in your 1-Day Food Record. If there is a food or product you ate that is *not* listed in the table, use the sodium value of the most similar food or, if it's a product, use the amount of sodium listed on the nutrition information label on the package.

Step 2

Total up how much sodium you consumed during the day. Was it more or less than 2,400 milligrams? Remember, this total doesn't include any salt, Ac'cent, seasoning salts, or soy sauce that you may have added at the table.

Step 3

Now use Table 10.4 to add up the total grams of sugar contained in the foods you listed in your 1-Day Food Record. If a food or product you ate is *not* listed in the table, use the sugar content of the most similar food, or use the amount of sugar listed on the package label. Many products, in compliance with the new food labeling law, now list their sugar content on the nutrition information label.

Step 4

Total up how much sugar you consumed during the day, and multiply the total number of grams by 4. This is how many calories from sugar you consumed. To

Table 10.4   Sugar Contents of Common Foods

Food Source and Serving Size	Sugar (g)
Cakes and Brownies	
Angel food cake, 1 piece	24.0
Brownie with nuts	25.0
Carrot cake, with cream cheese icing, 1 piece	38.0
Chocolate cake, with vanilla icing, 1 piece	48.0
Chocolate cupcake, with chocolate icing	21.0
Lemon cake, with icing (two-layer), 1 piece	67.0
Pound cake, 1 piece	15.0
Yellow cake, with chocolate icing, 1 piece	26.0
Cookies	
Chocolate chip cookie	4.0
Cinnamon coffee cake, with crumb topping, 1 piece (63 g)	19.0
Muffin, blueberry, medium	6.0
Muffin, bran, homemade	7.0
Oatmeal raisin cookie	5.0
Peanut butter cookie	5.0
Reduced-fat sandwich cookie	4.0
Sandwich cookie, all types	4.0
Snickerdoodle cookie	6.0
Sweet roll	12.0
Beverages	
Fruit-flavored soda, 1 cup	28.0
Ginger ale, 1 cup	21.0
Hot chocolate/cocoa mix, 1 packet	21.5
Iced tea, sweetened, 1 cup	22.0
Instant breakfast powder, 1 envelope	24.0
Kool-Aid-type, 1 cup	23.0
Lemonade, 1 cup	23.0
Lemonade, pink, 1 cup	23.0
Liqueurs	
Amaretto, kahlua, 1 shot	12.0
Coffee liqueur, 1 oz	11.0
Creme de menthe, 1 oz	12.0
Triple sec, sloe gin, 1 shot	12.0
	(continued next page)

Table 10.4. (continued)

Food Source and Serving Size	Sugar (g)
Ovaltine malted milk powder, 1 oz	11.5
Punch, 1 cup	30.0
Soda	
Cola-type, 1 cup	26.0
Root beer, 1 cup	26.0
7UP-type, 1 cup	26.0
Tonic water, 1 cup	21.0
Candy	
Caramels, 2 pieces	12.1
Chocolate-covered mint patties, 2	17.2
Chocolate-covered peanuts, ¼ cup	11.7
Chocolate-covered raisins, ¼ cup	29.0
Chocolate fudge, 2 pieces	25.8
Gumdrops, small, 8	24.5
Gummy bears, 8	24.5
Hard candy, 1 oz	27.6
Jelly beans, 1 oz	26.3
Lollipop, 1 oz	27.5
Candy Bars	
M & M's, 1.7 oz	27.0
Mars Almond Candy Bar	29.0
Milk chocolate candy bar	23.0
Milky Way	43.0
Mounds	29.0
Nestle Crunch, 2 oz	28.0
Reese's Peanut Butter Cups, 2	21.0
Skor English Toffee Candy Bar	12.0
Snickers, 2 oz	36.0
Twix, 1.8 oz	20.0
Cooking Extras	
Flaked coconut, sweetened, ½ cup	14.0
Marshmallows, miniature, ½ cup	18.4
Sweetened condensed milk, 4 oz	83.0
Fruits	
Apricots in heavy syrup, ½ cup	26.1
Blueberries in heavy syrup, canned, ½ cup	26.4

Table 10.4. (continued)

Food Source and Serving Size	Sugar (g)
Boysenberries in heavy syrup, ½ cup	25.2
Mixed fruit, frozen with sugar, ½ cup	27.9
Strawberry slices, frozen with sugar, ½ cup	30.6
Sweet cherries in heavy syrup, ½ cup	25.2
Frozen Desserts	
Banana split, with whipped cream	99.0
Chocolate ice cream (Breyers), ½ cup	19.3
Chocolate ice cream, soft-serve, ½ cup	23.1
Creamsicle/dreamsicle bar	17.4
Drumstick ice cream bar	13.8
English toffee ice cream bar (Heath)	17.1
Frozen yogurt, vanilla, ½ cup	13.0
Fruit sorbet, ½ cup	23.6
Fudgsicle ice cream bar	14.5
Ice cream bar with chocolate coating (Dove)	31.8
Ice cream cookie sandwich (Chipwich)	16.1
Ice cream sandwich	14.8
Low-fat praline ice cream (Healthy Choice), ½ cup	24.0
Low-fat vanilla ice cream (Healthy Choice), ½ cup	17.0
Orange sherbet, ½ cup	29.2
Popsicle	18.0
Premium ice milk, all flavors (Breyer's Light), ½ cup	18.5
Other Desserts	
Caramel/candy apple	52.0
Pudding (average of all flavors), ½ cup	16.0
Pies and Pastries	
Apple pie, ⅛ of 9″ pie	24.0
Blueberry pie, ⅛ of 9″ pie	20.0
Cherry pie, ⅛ of 9″ pie	30.0
Cherry crisp, 1 serving (3″ × 3″)	21.0
Doughnut, cake-type	8.0
Peach crisp, 1 serving (3″ × 3″)	24.0
Pop Tart, frosted	19.0
Pop Tart, fruit-filled	13.0

(continued next page)

Table 10.4. (continued)

Food Source and Serving Size	Sugar (g)
Snacks	
Banana chips, 1.5 oz	16.6
Granola bar, hard	9.0
Granola bar, hard, peanut	7.0
Granola bar, soft (chocolate-coated)	17.0
Twinkie (42 g)	25.0
Table Extras	
Apple butter, 2 Tbsp	16.0
Catsup, 1 Tbsp	4.0
Chocolate syrup, 2 Tbsp	19.0
Cool Whip dessert topping, ½ cup	9.0
Cranberry sauce, canned, ½ cup	52.5
Dream Whip dessert topping, ½ cup	5.5
Jam, 1 Tbsp	14.0
Jelly, 1 Tbsp	12.5
Honey, 1 Tbsp	17.0
Hot fudge chocolate topping, 2 Tbsp	19.0
Molasses, light, 1 Tbsp	11.0
Pancake syrup, 1 Tbsp	9.0
Pancake syrup, light, 1 Tbsp	4.5
Peanut butter, 2 Tbsp	5.0
Sugar, granulated, 1 Tbsp	12.0
Yogurt	
Fruit on the bottom-type yogurt, 1 cup	44.0
Low-fat flavored yogurt, 1 cup	34.0
Low-fat fruit yogurt, 1 cup	30.0
Nonfat fruit yogurt, with Nutrasweet, 1 cup	14.0

get your percent of calories from sugar, divide the number of calories from sugar by the total number of calories you consumed during the day, and multiply the result by 100.

Are you getting about 10 percent or less of your calories from sugar? Or are you getting far more sugar?

APPENDIX A
NUTRITION TABLES

Table A.1. Best Food Sources of Lignans*

Food Source	Total Lignans Provided[+]	Food Source	Total Lignans Provided[+]
Oil Seeds		*Whole-Grain Cereals*	
Flaxseed meal	67,543	Triticale	924
Flaxseed flour	52,679	Wheat	490
Rapeseeds	1,130	Oats	340
Soybeans	863	Brown rice	297
Sunflower seeds	396	Sorghum	255
Peanuts	161	Corn	230
		Rye	160
Dried Seaweeds		Barley	115
Mekuba	1,147		
Hijiki	653	*Vegetables*	
		Garlic	407
Dried Whole Legumes		Squash	381
Lentils	1,787	Asparagus	374
Kidney beans	561	Carrot	346
Alfalfa seeds	498	Sweet potatoes	295
Navy beans	460	Broccoli	226
Fava beans	217	Leeks	198
Yellow peas	213	Green peppers	195
Pinto beans	203	Turnips	156
		Cauliflower	145
Cereal Brans		Beets	135
Oat bran	651	Snow peas	122
Corn bran	648	Iceberg lettuce	121
Wheat bran	567	Onions	112
Barley bran	383		
Rice bran	181	*Fruits*	
		Pears	181
		Plums	145

*The food category producing the highest average amount of lignans (oil seeds) is listed first, followed by the second-highest category (dried seaweeds), and so forth, with the specific foods producing the highest amounts listed in order within each category.

[+]Enterolactone and enterodiol, in µg per 3½ oz of food.

Table A.2.   Best Food Sources of Isoflavonoids*

Apples
Berries
Broccoli
Cabbage
Carrots
Citrus fruits
Cucumbers
Eggplant
Garlic
Grapes
Lettuce (all types)
Parsley
Peppers (all types)
Soy Products
Squash (all types)
Strawberries
Tomatoes
Yams

*Although studies have shown these foods to be high in isoflavonoids, exact amounts are not currently available. For convenience, they are listed here in alphabetical order.

Table A.3. Best Food Sources of Boron

Food Sources	Boron Content (mg per 100 g of dried food)*	Food Sources	Boron Content (mg per 100 g of dried food)*
Fruits and Vegetables		Black beans (fruits and seeds)	4.5
Plums (prunes when dried)	25.5	Spinach	4.0
Quinces	16.0	Carrots	3.6
Strawberries	16.0	Grapefruit	3.3
Peaches	15.0	Rutabaga (roots)	3.0
Cabbage	14.5	Butter beans	3.0
Dandelion (leaves)	12.5	Oranges	2.8
Apples	11.0	Rutabaga (stems)	2.4
Asparagus	10.4	Endive	2.4
Celery (roots)	10.3	Peas (seeds)	2.3
Figs	10.0	Broccoli (stems)	2.1
Tomatoes	9.6	Brussels sprouts (stems)	2.1
Lettuce	8.7	Chinese cabbage	2.1
Broccoli (leaves)	8.5	Turnip (roots)	2.0
Pears	8.2	Chicory (roots)	2.0
Beets	8.0	Sweet potatoes	2.0
Sour cherries	8.0	Cauliflower (stems)	1.8
Red currants	8.0	Bell peppers	1.8
Cauliflower (florets)	7.6	Soybeans	1.8
Apricots	7.0	Bananas	1.8
Radishes	6.4	Mangoes	1.8
Black currants	6.4	Cantaloupe	1.7
Celery (seeds)	6.1	Wheat (seeds)	1.6
Brussels sprouts (leaves)	5.7	Papaya	1.5
Cowpeas	5.7	Gooseberries	1.5
Rutabaga (leaves)	5.2	Corn	1.5
American persimmons	5.0	Mandarin oranges	1.4
Grapes	5.0	Avocados	1.3
Cucumbers	4.6	Red raspberries	1.3
Onions	4.5	Sesame seeds	1.3
Alfalfa sprouts	4.5	Blueberries	1.3

*Several different laboratories have published tables listing the boron content of various foods. However, the amounts may differ slightly because it is difficult to measure boron content exactly.

Source: James A. Duke, Economic Botanist, USDA (Agricultural Research Service).

Table A.4. Better Breakfast Cereals

Breakfast Cereal	Serving Size	Fiber (g)	Fat (g)	Percentage of Calories from Fat	Sugar (g)	Percentage of Calories from Sugar	Calcium (% Daily Value)*
Best Choices							
Quaker Oat Squares	1 cup	4	3.0	12%	9	16%	4%
Multi Bran Chex	1¼ cups	7	2.0	8%	11	20%	0%
Almond Delight	1 cup	4	3.0	13%	12	23%	2%
100% Whole Grain Wheat Chex	¾ cup	5	1.0	5%	5	11%	0%
Clusters	1 cup	4	4.5	18%	14	25%	16%
Blueberry Muesli	1 cup	4	2.5	11%	14	28%	30%
Raisin Nut Bran	1 cup	5	4.5	19%	15	29%	6%
Fiber One	½ cup	13	1.0	15%	0	0%	4%
Healthy Choice Multi Grain Squares	1¼ cups	6	1.0	5%	8	17%	0%
All Bran Extra Fiber	½ cup	15	1.0	18%	0	0%	10%
All Bran Original	½ cup	10	1.0	11%	5	25%	10%
Mueslix Golden Crunch	⅔ cup	6	5.0	21%	11	21%	4%
Nutri-Grain Golden Wheat	¾ cup	4	0.5	5%	6	24%	0%
Complete Bran Flakes	¾ cup	5	0.5	5%	6	24%	0%
Natural Bran Flakes	⅔ cup	6	0.5	5%	5	22%	0%
Fruit & Fibre Peaches-Almonds	1 cup	6	3.0	13%	15	29%	2%
Great Grains Raisin-Date-Pecan	⅔ cup	5	5.0	21%	13	25%	2%
Great Grains Crunchy Pecan	⅔ cup	4	6.0	25%	8	15%	2%
Grape Nuts	½ cup	5	0.0	0%	7	14%	2%

Banana Nut Crunch	1 cup	4	6.0	22%	11	18%	2%
Frosted Wheat Bites	1 cup	5	1.0	5%	11	23%	2%
Frosted Mini-Wheats	1 cup	6	1.0	5%	12	25%	0%
Bite Size Frosted Mini-Wheats	1 cup	6	1.0	5%	12	25%	0%
Raisin Squares	¾ cup	5	1.0	5%	12	27%	0%
Shredded Wheat 'n Bran	1½ cups	8	1.0	5%	1	2%	2%
Shredded Wheat Spoon Size	1 cup	5	0.5	3%	0	0%	2%
Shredded Wheat	2 biscuits	5	0.5	3%	0	0%	2%
Good Choices[+]							
Total Raisin Bran	1 cup	5	1.0	5%	20	44%	20%
Healthy Choice Raisin & Crunchy	1¼ cups	4	2.0	9%	16	32%	2%
Clusters							
Mueslix Raisin & Date Crispy Blend	⅔ cup	4	3.0	14%	16	32%	2%
Nutri-Grain Almond Raisin	1¼ cups	4	3.0	14%	16	32%	2%
Nutri-Grain Golden Wheat & Raisins	1¼ cups	6	1.0	3%	18	40%	2%
Fruit & Fibre Dates & Walnuts	1 cup	6	3.0	13%	18	34%	2%
100% Bran	⅓ cup	8	0.5	6%	7	35%	2%
Kellogg's Raisin Bran	1 cup	7	1.0	5%	19	45%	2%
Post Raisin Bran	1 cup	8	1.0	5%	20	42%	2%

*A new term used on nutrition information labels, which in most cases is equivalent to RDA.

[+]The cereals listed here may have a bit more sugar than those listed under "Best Choices," but they offer many of the same nutritional benefits, including good fiber content, little fat, and some calcium.

Table A.5.   Product Choices to Cut Sugar Consumption*

Pancake Syrup
Cary's Low Calorie Syrup
S & W Nutradiet Strawberry and Maple Syrup

Puddings/Gelatin Desserts
D-Zerta Sugar Free Puddings
D-Zerta Sugar Free Low Calorie Gelatin Dessert
Estee Reduced Calorie Instant Pudding/Pie Filling
Jell-O Sugar Free Instant Pudding/Pie Filling
Jello-O Sugar Free Gelatin Dessert
Sans Sucre de Paris (Cheesecake Mousse, Chocolate Mousse)

Hot Cocoa Mixes
Carnation Hot Cocoa No Sugar Added
Carnation Hot Cocoa Fat Free
Swiss Miss Sugar Free

Other Beverages
Crystal Light low calorie beverages, assorted flavors

Yogurt
Dannon Light (sweetened with Nutrasweet); 8 oz provides 100 calories, 0 g of fat,
    and 14 g of sugar (strawberry).
Yoplait Light (sweetened with Nutrasweet and fructose); 6 oz provides 90 calories,
    0 g of fat, and 8 g of sugar.

Ice Cream and Frozen Desserts
Dreyer's Grand No Sugar Added
Eskimo Pie No Sugar Added (but still high in fat); 1 bar provides 150 calories, 11 g
    of fat, and 3 g of sugar.
Nestle Crunch Reduced Fat Dessert Bar (but still contains some fat); 1 bar provides
    130 calories, 7 g of fat, and 6 g of sugar.
Klondike Lite Dessert Bar (but still contains some fat); 1 bar provides 110 calories,
    6 g of fat, and 14 g of carbohydrate (sugar values were not available).
Sugar Free Fudgsicle; 1 bar provides 35 calories and 1 g of fat.
Welch's Light Fruit Juice Bars; 1 bar provides 25 calories, 0 g of fat, and 6 g of sugar.
Dole No Sugar Added Juice Bars; 1 bar provides 25 calories, 0 g of fat, and 3 g of
    sugar.

Pancake Syrup
Log Cabin Lite, 50% less calories
Eggo Lite, 60% less calories
Aunt Jemima Lite and Butter Lite, 50% less calories
Mrs. Butterworth's Lite, 45% less calories

Jams / Preserves
Smucker's Low Sugar (half the sugar)
Smucker's Light (66% fewer calories than regular); contains fructose, sugar, and
    Nutrasweet.

---

*Most of these products are sweetened with Nutrasweet or other artificial
    sweeteners. Some may still contain some sugar.

Table A.5. (continued)

Knott's Light (60% fewer calories than regular); contains high-fructose corn syrup and Nutrasweet.

Canned/Bottled Fruits

Applesauce, no sugar added (Seneca 100% Natural, Mott's Natural, Apple Time Original Unsweetened, Tree Top Natural)

Fruit Cocktail, canned in juice (Libby's Lite, Del Monte Fruit Naturals, S & W)

Grapefruit, canned in juice (S & W)

Mixed fruit, canned in juice (Del Monte Fruit Naturals)

Peaches, canned in juice (Libby's Lite, S & W Natural Style, Del Monte Fruit Naturals)

Pears, canned in juice (Libby's Lite, Del Monte Fruit Naturals)

Pineapple, canned in juice (Del Monte Fruit Naturals, Dole)

The following are canned in water:

S & W Nutradiet (pineapple, mandarin oranges, apricot halves, peach slices, pear halves, fruit cocktail, grapefruit sections, and applesauce).

The following are canned with the sweetener sodium saccharin:

S & W Nutradiet (pear halves and quarters, whole plums, fruit cocktail, sliced peaches, peach halves, and whole apricots).

Table A.6. Calories, Fat, Protein, and Sodium

Food and Serving Size	Calories	Fat (g)	Protein (g)	Sodium (mg)
Breads and Cereals				
Breads				
Bagel, cinnamon raisin	155	1.0	6.0	183
Bagel, egg	189	1.0	7.0	344
Bagel, whole wheat	143	1.0	6.0	269
Bread crumbs, dry, 1 oz	112	1.5	4.0	244
Bun, hamburger	129	2.0	4.0	252
Bun, hot dog	114	2.0	3.0	224
Cornbread, 1 piece	176	5.0	4.0	427
Date-nut bread, 1 piece	216	10.0	3.0	140
Dinner roll, french	105	1.6	3.0	232
English muffin	134	1.0	4.0	265
English muffin, cinnamon and raisin	139	1.5	4.0	255
French bread, 1 piece	96	1.0	3.0	213
Pita pocket, 1 piece	165	0.7	5.0	321
Pumpernickel bread, 1 piece	80	1.0	3.0	214
Raisin bread, 1 piece	69	1.0	2.0	98
Sourdough bread, 1 piece	69	0.8	2.0	152
White bread, 1 piece	91	1.3	3.0	163
Whole-wheat bread, 1 piece	86	1.5	3.0	184
Cold Cereals				
All Bran, ½ cup	107	0.8	6.0	486
Alpha Bits, 1 cup	111	0.7	2.0	180

(continued next page)

Table A.6.   (continued)

Food and Serving Size	Calories	Fat (g)	Protein (g)	Sodium (mg)
Apple Jacks, 1 cup	110	0.0	2.0	125
Bran Buds, ½ cup	111	1.0	6.0	265
Bran Chex, ½ cup	78	0.7	3.0	227
Bran flakes, 1 cup	127	0.7	5.0	303
Cap'n Crunch, 1 cup	156	3.4	2.0	278
Cheerios, 1 cup	89	1.5	3.0	246
Cheerios, Honey Nut, 1 cup	125	0.8	4.0	299
Corn flakes, 1 cup	97	0.0	2.0	256
Crispix, 1 cup	110	0.0	2.0	220
Frosted Flakes, 1 cup	144	0.0	2.0	306
Golden Grahams, 1 cup	150	1.5	2.0	386
Grape Nuts, ½ cup	195	0.2	6.0	379
Grape Nut Flakes, 1 cup	140	0.4	4.0	220
Just Right with fiber nuggets, ½ cup	76	0.8	2.0	152
Just Right with fruit and nuts, ½ cup	93	0.7	2.0	127
Kix, 1 cup	74	0.4	2.0	193
Life, 1 cup	163	0.8	8.0	230
Mueslix crispy blend, ½ cup	114	1.5	2.0	114
Mueslix golden crunch, ½ cup	120	1.0	3.0	170
Nature Valley Granola, ½ cup	251	9.8	6.0	116
Product 19, 1 cup	126	0.2	3.0	378
Raisin Bran, ½ cup	87	0.6	3.0	155
Rice Chex, 1 cup	99	0.0	1.0	210
Rice Krispies, 1 cup	111	0.0	2.0	206
Shredded Wheat, ½ cup	77	0.5	2.0	2
Special K, 1 cup	110	0.0	6.0	265
Total Wheat, 1 cup	116	0.7	3.0	326
Wheat Chex, ½ cup	85	0.6	2.0	154
Wheaties, 1 cup	101	0.5	3.0	276
Hot Cereals				
Malt O Meal, ½ cup	61	0.0	2.0	1
Oatmeal, 1 cup	145	2.3	6.0	2
Roman Meal, ½ cup	74	0.5	3.0	1
Pastries				
Cake doughnut	211	11.4	3.0	273
Cheese danish	265	15.5	6.0	319
Chocolate doughnut with icing	272	16.0	4.0	129
Cinnamon danish	354	20.0	6.0	325
Fruit danish	263	13.0	4.0	251
Jelly-filled doughnut	221	12.0	4.0	190
Pop Tart	212	5.5	3.0	226
Raised doughnut	241	13.7	4.0	205

Table A.6. (continued)

Food and Serving Size	Calories	Fat (g)	Protein (g)	Sodium (mg)
Grains				
Pasta: (½-cup cooked servings)				
Macaroni, whole-wheat	87	0.4	4.0	2
Rotini	99	0.5	3.0	1
Small shells	81	0.4	3.0	1
Spaghetti	115	0.2	6.0	4
Spirals	95	0.4	3.0	1
Vermicelli	99	0.5	3.0	1
Rice (½-cup cooked servings)				
Brown rice	108	0.9	3.0	5
Flavored rice and pasta (Rice A Roni)	133	3.0	3.0	619
Fried rice, meatless	120	5.8	2.0	141
Spanish rice	104	1.7	2.0	335
White rice	133	0.3	3.0	1
White rice, instant	81	0.1	2.0	2
Wild rice	83	0.3	3.0	2
Beans (½-cup servings unless otherwise noted)				
Baby lima beans, boiled	115	0.3	7.0	3
Baked beans, homemade	190	6.5	7.0	531
Baked beans, vegetarian	118	0.6	6.0	504
Black beans, cooked with salt	114	0.5	8.0	204
Boston baked beans, fat-free, 3 oz	76	0.0	3.2	116
Broadbeans/fava beans, boiled	94	0.3	6.5	4
Garbanzo beans, canned	143	1.4	6.0	359
Kidney beans, boiled	112	0.4	7.6	2
Lima beans, canned	82	0.3	4.6	201
Navy beans, canned	148	0.6	10.0	586
Navy beans, cooked with salt	129	0.5	8.0	216
Northern beans, canned	149	0.5	9.7	5
Northern beans, cooked with salt	104	0.4	7.4	211
Pink beans, boiled	125	0.4	7.6	2
Pinto beans, cooked with salt	117	0.4	7.0	203
Pork and beans, canned	124	1.3	6.5	557
Refried beans, canned	135	1.4	8.0	537
White beans, boiled	127	0.6	8.0	2
Milk and Dairy Products				
Cheeses				
American cheese, 1 piece	79	6.6	5.0	300
American cheese, nonfat (KraftFree Singles), 1 piece	46	0.0	7.0	425
American Cheese Spread (Cheez Whiz), 1 oz	82	6.0	5.0	381

(continued next page)

Table A.6.   (continued)

Food and Serving Size	Calories	Fat (g)	Protein (g)	Sodium (mg)
Blue cheese, ½ oz	50	4.0	3.0	198
Brie cheese, 1 oz	95	8.0	6.0	178
Cheddar cheese, 1 oz	114	9.4	7.0	176
Feta cheese, 1 oz	75	6.0	4.0	316
Gorgonzola cheese, 1 oz	111	9.0	7.0	512
Gouda cheese, 1 oz	101	7.8	7.0	232
Monterey jack cheese, 1 oz	106	8.6	7.0	152
Mozzarella cheese, low-fat, 1 oz	79	5.0	8.0	150
Parmesan cheese, grated, ¼ cup	114	7.5	10.0	465
Provolone cheese, 1 oz	100	7.5	7.0	248
String cheese, 1 stick	72	4.5	7.0	132
Swiss cheese, 1 oz	107	7.8	8.0	74
Swiss cheese, low-fat, 1 oz	51	1.5	8.0	74
Milks				
Buttermilk, 8 oz	99	2.2	8.0	257
Chocolate milk, nonfat, 8 oz	144	1.2	9.0	121
Chocolate milk, 1% low-fat, 8 oz	158	2.5	8.0	152
Chocolate milk, 2% low-fat, 8 oz	179	5.0	8.0	151
Chocolate milk, whole, 8 oz	209	8.5	8.0	149
Evaporated nonfat milk, 4 oz	99	0.3	10.0	147
Evaporated 2% low-fat milk, 4 oz	116	2.5	9.0	142
Evaporated whole milk, 4 oz	169	9.5	9.0	134
Low-fat milk, 1%, 8 oz	102	2.6	8.0	123
Low-fat milk, 2%, 8 oz	121	4.7	8.0	122
Nonfat milk, 8 oz	86	0.4	8.0	126
Whole milk, 8 oz	150	8.0	8.0	120
Cream				
Creamer, powder, 1 tsp	11	0.7	0.0	4
Cream, half and half, 4 oz	157	14.0	4.0	49
Cream, heavy whipping, 4 oz	205	22.0	1.0	22
Cream, table/coffee, 4 oz	234	23.0	3.0	48
Cream, 25% fat, 4 oz	292	30.0	3.0	44
Nondairy creamer, 1 tsp	6	0.5	0.0	2
Whipped cream, pressurized, ½ cup	77	6.7	1.0	39
Whipping cream, light, whipped, ½ cup	174	18.5	1.0	21
Other Dairy Products				
Cream cheese, 1 oz	99	10.0	2.0	84
Cream cheese, low-fat, ¼ cup	139	10.6	6.0	178
Cream cheese, nonfat, ¼ cup	100	0.0	16.0	682
Cottage cheese, low- sodium, low-fat, ½ cup	81	1.0	14.0	15
Cottage cheese, nonfat, 4 oz	70	0.0	15.0	422
Cottage cheese, 1% low-fat, ½ cup	82	1.2	14.0	459

Table A.6. (continued)

Food and Serving Size	Calories	Fat (g)	Protein (g)	Sodium (mg)
Cottage cheese, 2% low-fat, ½ cup	101	2.0	16.0	459
Creamed cottage cheese, ½ cup	108	4.8	13.0	425
Light Neufchatel Cheese, 1 oz	81	7.0	3.0	117
Ricotta cheese, part skim, ½ cup	170	9.7	14.0	154
Sour cream, 2 Tbsp	62	6.0	1.0	15
Sour cream, imitation, 2 Tbsp	60	5.6	1.0	29
Sour cream, low-calorie, 2 Tbsp	41	3.6	1.0	12
Sour cream, nonfat, 2 Tbsp	18	0.0	2.0	20
Yogurt (½ cup servings)				
Yogurt, low-fat, custard-style, fruit flavor	125	1.3	5.0	72
Yogurt, low-fat, fruit	125	1.3	5.0	72
Yogurt, low-fat, plain	78	1.9	6.0	86
Yogurt, nonfat, plain	68	0.2	7.0	94
Yogurt whole milk, plain	75	4.0	4.0	57
Desserts (1-piece servings unless otherwise noted)				
Angel food cake	137	0.4	3.0	397
Applesauce cake with nuts and icing	399	13.3	3.0	293
Banana cake with icing	309	7.6	3.5	292
Carrot cake with cream cheese icing	488	30.0	5.0	276
Cheesecake, 1/12 of 9" cake	457	33.3	9.0	362
Chocolate cake with chocolate icing	253	11.0	3.0	230
Chocolate cupcake with chocolate icing	154	7.0	2.0	140
Coffee cake, cheese	258	11.6	5.0	258
Coffee cake, cinnamon with crumb topping	263	14.7	4.0	221
Cookies (1 unless otherwise noted)				
Animal crackers/cookies, 5	51	1.6	1.0	45
Butter	23	1.0	0.3	18
Chocolate-chip, from recipe	49	3.0	1.0	36
Chocolate sandwich, cream-filled	47	2.0	0.5	61
Fig bar	49	1.0	0.5	49
Fig Newton, fat-free	68	0.0	1.0	76
Fortune	30	0.2	0.3	22
Fudge cookie, cake-type	73	0.8	1.0	40
Gingersnap	29	0.7	0.4	46
Macaroon	97	3.0	1.0	59
Oatmeal raisin	57	2.0	1.0	70
Peanut butter, from recipe	57	3.0	1.0	62
Pecan sandies	75	3.5	1.0	9
Shortbread	40	2.0	0.5	37
Snickerdoodle	81	3.5	1.0	68
Vanilla wafer	18	0.6	0.2	13
Frozen yogurt, chocolate, low-fat, ½ cup	110	2.0	5.0	57

(continued next page)

Table A.6. (continued)

Food and Serving Size	Calories	Fat (g)	Protein (g)	Sodium (mg)
Frozen yogurt, chocolate, nonfat, ½ cup	104	0.8	5.5	62
Frozen yogurt, vanilla with fruit, nonfat, ½ cup	96	0.2	5.0	65
Frozen yogurt, vanilla, soft-serve, ½ cup	114	4.0	3.0	63
Fruitcake	155	5.0	2.0	62
German chocolate cake with icing	404	21.0	4.0	369
Ice cream, chocolate, ½ cup	160	8.0	3.0	30
Ice cream cookie sandwich (Chipwich)	144	5.6	3.0	36
Ice cream, strawberry, ½ cup	130	6.0	2.0	40
Ice cream, vanilla, ½ cup	133	7.3	2.0	53
Ice cream, vanilla, soft-serve, ½ cup	185	11.2	3.5	36
Lemon cake with icing, 2-layer	388	11.3	3.0	248
Pies (⅛ of 9″ pie)				
Apple	301	14.2	3.0	239
Banana cream	305	15.4	5.0	272
Blackberry	303	14.0	3.0	221
Blackbottom	318	19.0	6.0	179
Blueberry	278	13.5	3.0	210
Cherry	306	13.8	3.0	217
Chocolate chiffon	367	18.3	7.0	211
Chocolate cream	320	18.2	5.0	278
Coconut cream	338	18.0	5.0	304
Egg custard	234	10.0	6.0	229
Grasshopper	379	20.3	5.5	545
Lemon meringue	323	14.6	4.0	274
Mincemeat	328	12.3	3.0	288
Pecan	467	25.2	5.5	297
Pumpkin	231	10.5	5.0	255
Sweet potato	235	12.6	5.0	145
Pineapple upside-down cake	367	14.0	4.0	367
Poppyseed cake, without icing	354	17.5	7.0	251
Popsicle, vanilla pudding	75	2.0	2.0	50
Pound cake, made with butter, 1 thin piece	113	5.8	2.0	115
Puddings (½-cup servings)				
Bread with raisins	212	7.4	7.0	291
Chocolate, made with 2% low-fat milk, instant	150	2.8	5.0	417
Chocolate, made with milk (homemade)	221	5.7	5.0	137
Low-calorie, made with milk (D-Zerta)	88	2.4	4.0	303
Rice, made from mix, with 2% low-fat milk	161	2.3	5.0	158
Rice, with raisins, homemade	217	4.3	5.5	85
Tapioca, made with milk (homemade)	103	3.6	4.0	157
Tapioca, made with 2% low-fat milk	147	2.4	4.0	172

Table A.6. (continued)

Food and Serving Size	Calories	Fat (g)	Protein (g)	Sodium (mg)
Pudding (continued)				
Vanilla, made with milk (homemade)	130	4.0	4.0	113
Vanilla, made with 2% low-fat milk	148	2.4	4.0	406
Sponge cake	187	2.7	5.0	144
White cake with white icing	266	9.6	2.0	166
Yellow cake with chocolate icing	262	12.0	3.0	233
Eggs and Egg Dishes				
Egg, boiled	78	5.3	6.0	62
Egg, deviled (½ egg and filling)	62	5.0	4.0	94
Egg, fried in margarine, 1 large	92	7.0	6.0	163
Egg, scrambled with milk and margarine	101	7.4	7.0	171
Egg white, 1 large	17	0.0	4.0	55
Egg yolk, 1 large	60	5.0	3.0	7
Nonfat egg substitute, ¼ cup	30	0.0	6.0	100
Omelet, plain, 1 large egg	90	6.8	6.0	160
Omelet, Spanish, 1 egg	123	8.8	5.4	251
Omelet, with cheese and ham, 1 egg	142	10.8	10.0	369
Omelet, with sausage and mushroom, 1 egg	173	13.5	11.0	455
Quiche Lorraine, ⅛ of 9″ pie	540	43.5	15.0	567
Fats and Oils				
Blue Bonnet Spread, 1 Tbsp	102	11.5	0.0	127
Butter, 1 Tbsp	102	11.5	0.0	117
Butter, unsalted, 1 Tbsp	102	11.5	0.0	2
Corn, safflower, soybean, or canola oil, 1 Tbsp	120	13.6	0.0	0
Fleischmann's Light Margarine (tub), 1 Tbsp	65	7.3	0.0	70
Margarine, diet spread, 1 Tbsp	49	5.5	0.0	50
Margarine, hard (stick), 1 Tbsp	102	11.4	0.0	134
Margarine, liquid, 1 Tbsp	102	11.4	0.3	110
Olive oil, 1 Tbsp	119	13.5	0.0	0
Shortening, vegetable, 1 Tbsp	113	12.8	0.0	0
Touch of Butter Spread, 1 Tbsp	53	6.0	0.0	110
Frozen Dinners (1 unless otherwise noted)				
Armour				
Classic Chicken and Noodle Dinner	280	9.0	19.0	550
Classic Chicken Mesquite	280	13.0	21.0	630
Classic Chicken Parmigiana	360	18.0	24.0	1,202
Lite Beef Pepper Steak Dinner	210	4.0	16.0	870
Lite Chicken Burgundy Dinner	210	5.0	20.0	760
Lite Sweet and Sour Chicken	220	1.0	16.0	520

(continued next page)

Table A.6. (continued)

Food and Serving Size	Calories	Fat (g)	Protein (g)	Sodium (mg)
Banquet				
Beef Dinner	240	7.0	26.0	660
Fried Chicken Dinner	470	27.0	21.0	960
Healthy Choice				
Beef Pepper Steak Oriental	250	4.0	19.0	470
Breast of Turkey Dinner	280	3.0	22.0	460
Cacciatore Chicken	260	3.0	22.0	510
Chicken Parmigiana Dinner	300	1.5	23.0	490
Fettucini Alfredo Entree	240	5.0	9.0	430
Fiesta Chicken Fajitas	260	4.0	21.0	410
Glazed Chicken Entree	200	1.5	17.0	480
Honey Mustard Chicken	260	2.0	21.0	550
Sweet and Sour Chicken Dinner	310	5.0	23.0	250
Lean Cuisine				
Cheese Ravioli	250	8.0	12.0	500
Chicken and Vegetable	240	5.0	19.0	520
Chicken Enchiladas	220	6.0	13.0	390
Chicken Fettucini	270	6.0	22.0	580
Chicken Parmesan	220	5.0	22.0	530
Chicken Pie	320	10.0	18.0	590
Fettucini Alfredo	270	7.0	13.0	590
French Bread Pepperoni Pizza	330	7.0	20.0	590
Lasagna with Meat Sauce	270	6.0	19.0	560
Oriental Beef with Veggies and Rice	240	8.0	13.0	461
Roasted Turkey Breast	290	4.0	16.0	530
Spaghetti with Meat Sauce	290	6.0	14.0	550
Le Menu				
Ham Steak Dinner	292	10.0	19.0	1,491
Stouffer's Entree				
Beef Ravioli	370	14.0	17.0	680
Cheese Ravioli and Tomato Sauce	360	14.0	16.0	720
Chicken a la King	320	10.0	15.0	750
Chicken Divan	210	10.0	21.0	570
Chicken Enchilada	370	14.0	16.0	970
Lasagna and Meat	360	13.0	27.0	780
Macaroni with Beef	340	12.0	19.0	1,530
Pepperoni and Mushroom Pizza	430	21.0	17.0	1,000
Weight Watchers				
Beef Enchiladas Ranchero	190	5.0	18.0	500
Chicken Fettucini	280	9.0	22.0	590
Fried Fillet of Fish	230	8.0	5.0	450
Lasagna with Meat Sauce	270	6.0	24.0	510

Table A.6. (continued)

Food and Serving Size	Calories	Fat (g)	Protein (g)	Sodium (mg)
Fruits and Vegetables				
Fruits				
Apple, medium, with peel	81	0.5	0.0	0
Apple slices, ½ cup	33	0.2	0.0	0
Banana	105	0.5	1.0	1
Blackberries, ½ cup	38	0.3	0.5	0
Blueberries, ½ cup	41	0.3	0.5	4
Boysenberries, ½ cup	38	0.3	0.5	0
Cantaloupe, ½ cup	28	0.2	1.0	7
Casaba melon, ½ cup	30	0.1	0.0	9
Cherries, sweet, ½ cup	52	0.7	1.0	0
Cranberries, ½ cup	23	0.1	0.0	0
Grapefruit sections, ½ cup	37	0.2	1.0	0
Grapes, ½ cup	57	0.5	1.0	2
Honeydew melon, ½ cup	30	0.1	0.0	9
Kiwifruit	46	0.3	1.0	4
Mandarin oranges, canned, ½ cup	47	0.0	1.0	6
Melon balls (mixed), ½ cup	29	0.2	1.0	27
Nectarine	67	0.6	1.0	0
Nectarine slices, ½ cup	34	0.3	1.0	0
Orange, medium	62	0.2	1.0	0
Peach	37	0.0	1.0	0
Peach slices, ½ cup	37	0.0	1.0	0
Pear, medium	98	0.7	1.0	0
Pear slices, ½ cup	49	0.3	0.0	0
Pineapple chunks, fresh, ½ cup	38	0.3	0.0	1
Plum	36	0.4	0.5	0
Raspberries, ½ cup	30	0.3	0.5	0
Strawberries, sliced, ½ cup	25	0.3	0.5	1
Strawberries, whole, ½ cup	22	0.3	0.0	1
Watermelon, ½ cup	26	0.3	0.5	2
Fruit and Vegetable Juices				
Apple juice, bottled, 8 oz	117	0.3	0.0	7
Cranberry juice cocktail, 8 oz	144	0.3	0.0	5
Grape juice, bottled, 8 oz	154	0.2	1.0	8
Grapefruit juice, 8 oz	101	0.3	1.0	2
Orange juice, unsweetened, 8 oz	112	0.2	2.0	2
Pineapple juice, unsweetened, 8 oz	140	0.2	1.0	3
Prune juice, bottled, 8 oz	182	0.1	2.0	10
Tomato juice, canned, 8 oz	42	0.1	2.0	880
Tomato juice, low-sodium, canned, 8 oz	42	0.1	2.0	24
Vegetable juice (V-8), 8 oz	46	0.2	2.0	884
Vegetable juice (V-8), low-sodium, 8 oz	46	0.2	2.0	60

(*continued next page*)

Table A.6. (continued)

Food and Serving Size	Calories	Fat (g)	Protein (g)	Sodium (mg)
Vegetables (½-cup servings unless otherwise noted)				
Acorn squash, baked and mashed	69	0.2	1.0	5
Baby carrots, 5	19	0.3	0.4	18
Broccoli, boiled	22	0.3	2.0	20
Broccoli, cooked with cheese sauce	111	7.3	6.0	179
Broccoli, cooked with cream sauce	93	5.8	4.0	190
Broccoli florets, raw	12	0.2	1.0	12
Brussels sprouts, boiled	30	0.4	2.0	16
Butternut squash, baked and mashed	49	0.1	1.0	5
Cabbage, chopped, steamed	19	0.2	1.0	14
Cabbage, raw, shredded	9	0.1	0.5	6
Cabbage, red, raw	9	0.1	0.5	4
Carrot	31	0.1	1.0	25
Carrots, raw, grated	24	0.1	1.0	19
Carrot slices, steamed	34	0.1	1.0	27
Celery, 1 large outer stalk	6	0.1	0.3	35
Celery, raw, chopped	10	0.1	0.0	52
Chinese cabbage, steamed	11	0.2	1.0	55
Corn, boiled	89	1.0	2.7	14
Corn, 1 ear	117	1.0	3.9	5
Crookneck squash, boiled	18	0.3	1.0	1
Green beans, boiled	22	0.2	1.2	2
Green beans, Italian-style, boiled from frozen	18	0.1	1.0	9
Greens				
Beet, boiled	20	0.1	2.0	174
Beet, raw, chopped	4	0.0	0.4	38
Chicory, raw, chopped	21	0.3	2.0	41
Collard, boiled	17	0.1	1.0	10
Collard, raw, chopped	6	0.0	0.3	4
Dandelion, boiled	17	0.3	1.0	23
Dandelion, raw, chopped	12	0.2	1.0	21
Dock/sorrel, cooked	10	0.3	1.0	2
Dock/sorrel, raw chopped	15	0.5	1.0	3
Mustard, boiled	11	0.2	2.0	11
Mustard, raw, chopped	7	0.0	1.0	7
Turnip, boiled	14	0.2	1.0	21
Turnip, raw, chopped	7	0.1	0.4	11
Hubbard squash, baked	60	0.7	3.0	10
Kale, boiled	21	0.3	1.0	15
Mushroom pieces, boiled	21	0.4	2.0	2
Mushroom pieces, canned	19	0.2	1.0	332
Mushroom pieces, raw	9	0.1	1.0	1
Parsnips, boiled	63	0.2	1.0	8

Table A.6. (continued)

Food and Serving Size	Calories	Fat (g)	Protein (g)	Sodium (mg)
Parsnips, raw slices	50	0.2	1.0	7
Peas, boiled from frozen	62	0.2	4.0	70
Peas, low-sodium, canned	59	0.3	4.0	2
Snow peas, boiled	34	0.2	3.0	3
Spaghetti squash, boiled	23	0.2	0.5	14
Spaghetti squash, boiled or baked, with salt	23	0.2	0.5	198
Split peas, boiled from dry	116	0.4	8.0	2
Split peas, cooked with salt	116	0.4	8.0	233
Summer squash slices, boiled	18	0.3	1.0	1
Summer squash slices, boiled with salt	18	0.3	1.0	213
Sweet potato, candied, ½ cup	134	3.0	1.0	69
Sweet potatoes, canned, mashed, ½ cup	129	0.3	3.0	96
Sweet potato, medium, without peel	117	0.1	2.0	11
Tomatoes, green, raw, chopped	22	0.2	1.0	12
Tomatoes, stewed, canned	33	0.2	1.0	324
Tomatoes, stewed, low-sodium	33	0.2	1.0	20
Tomatoes, sun-dried, packed in oil, drained, 1 oz	60	4.0	1.0	75
Tomato, fried green	238	18.0	4.0	243
Tomato, ripe	26	0.4	1.0	11
Turnip cubes, boiled	14	0.1	1.0	39
Turnip cubes, raw	18	0.1	1.0	44
Wax beans, canned	14	0.1	0.8	169
Winter squash, baked and mashed	47	0.8	1.0	1
Winter squash, made with fat and sugar	97	3.0	1.0	295
Zucchini, boiled	14	0.0	1.0	3
Zucchini squash, raw	9	0.1	1.0	2
Lettuce (½ cup servings)				
Butter, chopped	4	0.0	0.4	1
Green leaf, chopped	5	0.0	0.4	3
Iceberg, chopped	4	0.0	0.3	3
Romaine, chopped	5	0.0	0.5	2
Potatoes				
Baked potato with skin, long	220	0.2	5.0	16
Baked potato with skin, medium	133	0.1	3.0	10
Cottage fries, oven-heated with salt, ½ cup	185	7.0	3.0	239
French fries, from frozen, ½ cup	90	4.7	1.0	62
Hash brown potatoes, ½ cup	119	10.8	2.0	19
Hash browns, fast-food serving	136	8.3	2	262
Mashed potatoes, made with whole milk and margarine, ½ cup	124	6.2	2.0	365

(*continued next page*)

Table A.6.   (continued)

Food and Serving Size	Calories	Fat (g)	Protein (g)	Sodium (mg)
Scalloped potatoes, ½ cup	105	4.5	4.0	411
Tater tots, ½ cup	138	6.6	2.0	463

Meat and Poultry

Beef (3-oz cooked servings unless otherwise noted)

Food and Serving Size	Calories	Fat (g)	Protein (g)	Sodium (mg)
Bottom round, lean, braised	187	8.0	27.0	43
Chuck roast, lean and fat, braised	282	20.0	23.0	51
Corned beef, cooked, trimmed	213	16.2	16.0	964
Filet mignon, trimmed, broiled	179	8.5	24.0	54
Flank steak, lean, broiled	176	8.6	23.0	71
Ground beef, extra-lean	224	13.6	24.0	69
London broil, trimmed, broiled	176	8.6	23.0	71
Porterhouse, lean and fat, broiled	259	18.8	21.0	52
Porterhouse, lean, broiled	185	9.2	24.0	56
Pot roast, lean and fat, roasted	234	14.0	24.0	43
Rib-eye steak, trimmed, broiled	191	9.9	24.0	59
Round eye, lean, roasted	149	4.9	25.0	53
Round steak, lean and fat, roasted	205	12.0	23.0	50
Rump roast, lean and fat, braised	220	12.8	25.0	43
Rump roast, lean only, braised	167	5.8	27.0	43
Short ribs, lean, braised	251	15.4	26.0	49
Short ribs, with sauce	255	20.6	11.0	356
Sirloin steak, lean, broiled	172	6.8	26.0	56
Stew meat, lean	199	9.6	27.0	253
T-bone, lean and fat, broiled	253	18.0	21.0	52
T-bone, lean only, broiled	182	8.9	24.0	56
Tenderloin steak, lean, broiled	179	8.5	24.0	54
Top round, lean, broiled	153	4.2	27	52
Top sirloin, lean and fat, broiled	241	15.6	23.0	53

Lamb (4-oz cooked servings)

Food and Serving Size	Calories	Fat (g)	Protein (g)	Sodium (mg)
Loin chop, lean only	245	11.0	34.0	95
Loin chop, with visible fat	357	26.2	28.5	87
Rib roast, lean only	263	15.0	30.0	92
Rib roast, with visible fat	407	33.8	24.0	83
Leg of lamb, with visible fat	292	18.7	29.0	75
Leg of lamb, lean only, roasted	216	8.8	32.0	77

Pork (4-oz cooked servings)

Food and Serving Size	Calories	Fat (g)	Protein (g)	Sodium (mg)
Loin center chop, broiled, lean only	261	12.0	36.0	89
Loin chop, braised, lean only	309	16.6	37.0	85
Loin chop, broiled, with visible fat	357	25.0	31.0	79
Pork center rib chop, lean only	277	15.7	32.0	52
Pork center rib chop, roasted, with visible fat	360	26.7	28.0	50
Pork leg, roasted, with visible fat	332	23.5	28.0	67

Table A.6. (continued)

Food and Serving Size	Calories	Fat (g)	Protein (g)	Sodium (mg)
Pork leg rump, roasted, lean only	249	12.0	33.0	74
Pork shoulder, braised, lean only	281	13.8	37.0	116
Pork shoulder, braised, with visible fat	391	29.0	30.0	100
Pork spareribs, with visible fat	450	34.3	33.0	105
Poultry (3-oz cooked servings, unless otherwise noted)				
Chicken breast, flour-fried	189	7.6	27.0	65
Chicken breast, fried, skinless	159	4.0	28.0	67
Chicken breast, roasted, with skin	168	6.6	25.0	60
Chicken breast, roasted, skinless	140	3.0	26.0	63
Chicken drumstick, flour-fried	208	12.0	23.0	76
Chicken drumstick, roasted	184	9.5	23.0	77
Chicken, fast-food serving, 2 pieces of dark meat	430	26.6	30.0	754
Chicken nuggets, fast-food serving	290	17.8	17.0	543
Chicken thigh, flour-fried	223	12.8	23.0	75
Chicken thigh, fried, skinless	185	9.0	24.0	81
Chicken thigh, roasted	210	13.2	21.0	71
Chicken thigh, roasted, skinless	178	9.3	22.0	75
Chicken wing, flour-fried	273	19.0	22.0	66
Chicken wing, roasted	247	16.6	23.0	70
Turkey, roasted, dark meat	188	9.8	23.0	65
Turkey, roasted, white meat	168	7.0	24.0	54
Lunch Meats and Meat Products (2-oz servings unless otherwise noted)				
Bacon, cooked, 2 strips	220	18.8	12.0	610
Bacon (Sizzlean), 2 strips	99	7.6	7.0	496
Bacon, turkey (Louis Rich), 2 strips	60	5.0	4.0	380
Beef lunch meat, thinly sliced	100	2.2	16.0	817
Bologna, beef	177	16.2	7.0	557
Bologna, Healthy Favorites	56	1.2	9.0	629
Bologna, turkey	113	8.6	8.0	497
Chicken breast, roasted, Deli Thin (Louis Rich)	65	1.6	10.0	676
Chicken or turkey breast, smoked lunch meat	62	1.0	13.0	811
Frankfurter, beef and pork	182	16.6	6.0	638
Frankfurter, chicken	116	8.8	6.0	617
Frankfurter (Healthy Favorites)	60	1.5	9.0	570
Frankfurter, turkey	102	8.0	6.0	642
Ham lunch meat, regular	103	6.0	10.0	747
Ham slices, extra-lean	74	2.8	11.0	810
Olive loaf	13	9.4	7.0	842
Polish sausage, pork	185	16.3	8.0	497
Polska kielbasa sausage, turkey	80	4.5	9.0	510

(continued next page)

Table A.6. (continued)

Food and Serving Size	Calories	Fat (g)	Protein (g)	Sodium (mg)
Roast beef, deli thin (Oscar Mayer)	65	1.6	12.0	578
Salami, beef	149	11.7	9.0	666
Salami, dry	237	19.5	13.0	1,055
Salami, turkey	111	7.8	9.0	569
Sausage links, pork, 2 (26 g)	96	8.0	5.0	336
Sausage patties, pork, 2 (54 g)	199	16.8	11.0	698
Turkey ham lunch meat, thigh	73	3.0	11.0	565
Mixed Dishes				
Burrito, bean	224	6.8	7.0	493
Burrito, bean and cheese	189	5.9	8.0	583
Burrito, beef	262	10.4	13.0	746
Burrito, breakfast (McDonald's)	290	17.0	12.0	580
Burrito, chicken (Taco Bell)	345	13.0	17.0	854
Burrito, 7-layer (Taco Bell)	485	21.0	15.0	1,115
Burrito supreme with red sauce (Taco Bell)	443	19.0	18.0	1,184
Chicken club sandwich (Wendy's)	520	25.0	30.0	990
Chicken fillet sandwich	515	29.5	24.0	957
Chicken or turkey noodle casserole, ½ cup	163	6.4	11.0	366
Chicken sandwich (BK Broiler)	540	29.0	30.0	480
Chicken sandwich on multigrain bun (Wendy's)	408	18.0	25.0	670
Chicken sandwich with cheese	632	38.8	29.0	1,238
Corn dog	460	19.0	17.0	973
Fajita, beef	409	17.5	17.0	850
Fajita, chicken	405	13.0	22.0	439
Filet-O-Fish sandwich (McDonald's)	364	16.2	14.0	708
Hamburger, double, with condiments	576	32.5	32.0	742
Hamburger, "Whopper" (Burger King)	630	39.0	27.0	850
Hamburger with condiments	275	10.2	14.0	564
Hot dog, chicken, on bun	235	11.0	9.0	819
Hot dog sandwich, plain	242	14.5	10.0	670
Hot dog, super size, 12" (Dairy Queen)	590	38.0	20.0	1,360
Hot Ham'n Cheese sandwich (Hardee's)	530	30.0	18.0	NA*
Lasagna, meatless, 1 serving	298	9.3	15.0	714
Lasagna, with meat, 1 serving	382	15.2	22.0	745
Macaroni and cheese, ½ cup	215	11.0	8.0	543
Roast beef sandwich, regular (Hardee's)	270	11.0	15.0	780
Spaghetti with clam sauce, ½ cup	229	10.0	13.0	218
Spaghetti with meatballs, ½ cup	166	6.0	9.0	505
Taco, beef, large	369	20.5	21.0	802
Taco, chicken	175	8.3	15.0	107
Taco salad (Jack in the Box)	470	23	34.0	1,470

*NA = Not available

Table A.6. (continued)

Food and Serving Size	Calories	Fat (g)	Protein (g)	Sodium (mg)
Tostada, bean and chicken	253	11.4	19.0	435
Tostada, beef and cheese	315	16.3	19.0	897
Tuna noodle casserole, ½ cup	119	3.7	8.0	388
Turkey club sandwich (Hardee's)	390	16.0	29.0	1,280
Nuts and Nut Products				
Almond butter, salted, 2 Tbsp	198	18.5	5.0	141
Almond butter, unsalted, 2 Tbsp	203	19.0	5.0	4
Filberts/hazelnuts, ½ cup	426	19.0	5.0	4
Macadamia nuts, dried, ½ cup	471	49.0	6.0	3
Mixed nuts, dry-roasted, ½ cup	407	35.5	12.0	458
Mixed nuts, dry-roasted, unsalted, ½ cup	407	35.5	12.0	8
Peanut butter, chunky, 2 Tbsp	188	16.0	8.0	156
Peanut butter, chunky, unsalted, 2 Tbsp	188	16.0	8.0	5
Peanut butter, smooth, 2 Tbsp	188	16.0	8.0	153
Peanut butter, smooth, unsalted, 2 Tbsp	191	16.8	9.0	5
Peanuts, dry-roasted, unsalted, ½ cup	427	36.0	17.0	4
Peanuts, oil-roasted, ½ cup	419	35.5	19.0	312
Pecans, dry-roasted, ½ cup	374	36.7	5.0	443
Pecans, dry-roasted, unsalted, ½ cup	390	38.2	5.0	1
Pine nuts, dried, 2 oz	292	28.7	14.0	2
Pistachios, dry-roasted, ½ cup	388	33.8	10.0	499
Soy nuts, ½ cup	190	10.0	16.0	2
Sunflower seed butter, 2 Tbsp	185	15.3	6.0	166
Tahini (sesame butter), 2 Tbsp	182	17.0	5.0	0
Walnuts, black, dried, chopped, ½ cup	379	35.4	15.0	1
Walnuts, English, dried, halved, ½ cup	321	31.0	7.0	5
Water chestnuts, canned, ½ cup	35	0.0	1.0	6
Salads (½-cup servings unless otherwise noted)				
Chicken salad with celery	268	24.7	11.0	201
Coleslaw	89	6.7	1.0	162
Coleslaw, fast-food serving	147	11.0	1.0	267
Macaroni salad, without cheese or egg	227	18.8	2.0	181
Potato salad, German	79	1.6	2.0	201
Potato salad, with mayonnaise and eggs	179	10.3	3.0	661
Potato salad, without egg	134	7.2	2.0	337
Shrimp salad	142	8.4	13.0	188
Tossed green salad	12	0.2	1.0	7
Tuna salad	192	9.5	16.0	412
Seafood				
Abalone, steamed or poached, ½ cup	157	1.0	26.0	384
Bluefish, baked or broiled, 4 oz	180	6.2	29.0	87
Bluefish, fried in crumbs, 4 oz	232	11.0	26.0	76

(continued next page)

Table A.6. (continued)

Food and Serving Size	Calories	Fat (g)	Protein (g)	Sodium (mg)
Crab, blue, canned, ½ cup	67	0.8	14.0	225
Crab cake	93	4.5	12.0	198
Crab, Dungeness, steamed or boiled, ½ cup	65	0.7	13.0	223
Crab, imitation, 3 oz	87	1.0	10.0	715
Crab, snow, baked or broiled, 3 oz	117	5.4	16.0	459
Crab, soft-shell, breaded and fried, 3 oz	284	17.0	17.0	439
Fish patty/square, 2	311	14.0	18.0	665
Fish sandwich, with cheese and tartar sauce	524	28.6	21.0	940
Fish sandwich, with tartar sauce	431	22.7	17.0	615
Fish sticks, heated from frozen, 4	310	14.0	18.0	663
Gefilte fish, sweet, 4 oz	95	2.0	10.0	594
Lobster, baked or broiled, ½ cup	84	2.2	14.0	450
Lobster tail, batter-fried, 3 oz	180	9.4	16.0	327
Lobster with butter sauce, ½ cup	224	17.7	15.0	452
Oysters, baked or broiled, ½ cup	62	1.6	7.0	210
Oysters, canned, ½ cup	86	3.0	9.0	139
Oysters, Eastern, breaded and fried, ½ cup	129	8.3	6.0	273
Pacific rockfish, baked or broiled, 4 oz	137	2.3	27.0	87
Prawns/large shrimp, steamed or broiled, 3 oz	84	1.0	18.0	191
Shrimp, batter-fried, ½ cup	158	8.0	13.0	295
Shrimp/prawns, breaded and fried, 3 oz	206	10.5	18.0	293
Shrimp, small, steamed or boiled, 3 oz	84	1.0	18.0	191
Squid/calamari, baked, ½ cup	97	3.3	13.0	259
Squid, flour-fried, ½ cup	131	5.6	13.0	229
Swordfish, baked or broiled, 4 oz	176	5.8	29.0	130
Whitefish, baked or broiled, 4 oz	195	8.5	28.0	74

Snacks

Chips (1-oz servings unless otherwise noted)

Corn chips	153	9.5	2.0	179
Potato chips	152	9.8	2.0	169
Potato chips, light	133	6.0	2.0	140
Potato chips, sour cream and onion	151	9.6	2.0	177
Pringles light chips	142	7.3	2.0	121
Tortilla chips (Doritos)	141	7.3	2.0	201
Tortilla chips, light	126	4.3	2.0	284

Crackers

Butter crackers (Club), 7	141	7.0	2.0	237
Butter crackers (Ritz), 10	151	7.6	2.0	254
Cheese crackers (Cheez-its), 30	151	8.0	3.0	299
Graham crackers, 4	118	3.0	2.0	169

Table A.6. (continued)

Food and Serving Size	Calories	Fat (g)	Protein (g)	Sodium (mg)
Matzoh cracker	112	0.4	3.0	1
100% Stoned Wheat crackers, 8	129	4.4	3.0	172
Saltines, 10	130	3.5	3.0	391
Wheat crackers (Wheat Thins), 10	143	6.7	2.0	261
Whole-grain rye crackers (Ry Krisp), 4	93	0.3	3.0	222
Whole-wheat crackers (Triscuits), 7	140	5.4	3.0	208
Granola Bars				
Fi-Bar, yogurt-coated granola bar	107	3.0	3.0	5
Hard granola bar	134	5.6	3.0	84
Soft granola bar	126	4.9	2.0	79
Soft granola bar, chocolate-chip, chocolate-coated	165	8.8	2.0	71
Soft granola bar, peanut butter, chocolate-coated	187	11.4	4.0	71
Other Snacks				
BBQ Cornuts, 3 oz	371	12.2	8.0	830
Caramel corn, 1 oz	122	3.6	1.0	58
Popcorn, air-popped, 1 oz	108	1.2	3.0	1
Popcorn, oil-popped, salted, 1 oz	142	8.0	2.5	251
Soups and Canned Entrees (½-cup servings unless otherwise noted)				
Bean and bacon soup, made with water	86	3.0	4.0	476
Beef stew	97	3.8	7.0	503
Bird's nest soup (chicken, ham, and noodles)	56	1.4	7.0	754
Black bean soup, made with water	58	0.8	3.0	599
Bouillabaisse soup/chowder	121	4.5	17.0	209
Chicken gumbo soup, made with water	28	0.7	1.0	477
Chicken noodle soup, made with water	37	1.2	2.0	553
Chicken rice soup, made with water	30	1.0	2.0	408
Chili and beans	143	7.0	7.0	666
Chili, vegetarian	144	7.6	8.0	417
Chunky chicken noodle soup	88	3.0	6.0	425
Chunky chicken rice soup	64	1.6	6.0	444
Chunky chicken vegetable soup	59	1.7	4.0	378
Chunky minestrone	64	1.4	3.0	432
Chunky split pea and ham soup	93	2.0	6.0	483
Chunky vegetable soup	61	1.9	2.0	505
Chunky turkey soup	68	2.2	5.0	462
Cream of broccoli soup	117	8.0	4.0	394
Cream of chicken soup, made with milk	96	5.8	4.0	523
Cream of mushroom soup, made with milk	102	6.8	3.0	538

(*continued next page*)

Table A.6. (continued)

Food and Serving Size	Calories	Fat (g)	Protein (g)	Sodium (mg)
Cream of mushroom soup, made with water	65	4.5	1.0	516
Cream of potato soup, made with milk	75	3.0	3.0	531
Cream of potato soup, made with water	37	1.2	1.0	500
Egg drop soup	37	2.0	4.0	365
Gazpacho soup, 3 oz	20	0.8	3.0	412
Lentil and ham soup	70	1.4	5.0	660
Low-sodium chicken vegetable soup	83	2.4	6.0	42
Low-sodium cream of mushroom soup	65	4.5	2.0	24
Low-sodium pea soup .	83	1.5	4.0	13
Low-sodium vegetable soup	41	1.2	1.0	21
Minestrone soup, made with water	41	1.3	2.0	456
Mushroom barley soup, made with water	37	1.0	1.0	446
Spaghetti sauce	136	6.0	2.0	618
Spaghetti sauce with meatballs	128	5.0	6.0	553
Split pea and ham soup, made with water	95	2.0	5.0	503
Tomato beef noodle soup, made with water	70	2.2	2.0	459
Tomato bisque soup, made with milk	99	3.3	3.0	555
Tomato bisque soup, made with water	62	1.3	1.0	524
Tomato rice soup, made with water	60	1.4	1.0	408
Tomato soup, made with milk	81	3.0	3.0	466
Tomato soup, made with water	43	1.0	1.0	436
Turkey vegetable soup, made with water	36	1.5	2.0	453
Vegetable beef soup, made with water	39	1.0	3.0	478
Vegetable soup, made with water	36	1.0	1.0	411
Wonton soup	94	3.5	7.0	380
Candy				
Butterfinger	286	11.4	4.0	121
Chocolate-coated peanuts, 1/2 cup	441	28.5	11.0	35
Milk chocolate bar	226	13.5	3.0	36
Milky Way	256	9.3	3.0	146
Snickers	267	13.0	6.0	157
3 Musketeers	251	7.8	2.0	117
Yogurt-covered peanuts, 1/2 cup	387	26.0	7.0	29
Beverages (see also "Fruit and Vegetable Juices")				
Alcoholic Beverages				
Beer, 12 oz	146	0.0	1.0	18
Beer, light, 12 oz	99	0.0	1.0	11
Gin, whiskey, brandy, rum, or vodka, 1 oz	75	0.0	0.0	1
Wine, red, 6 oz	127	0.0	0.4	9
Wine, white, 6 oz	120	0.0	0.2	9

Table A.6. (continued)

Food and Serving Size	Calories	Fat (g)	Protein (g)	Sodium (mg)
Soda (12-oz servings)				
Cola type	152	0.0	0.0	15
Cola type, caffeine-free	153	0.0	0.0	24
Cream soda	189	0.0	0.0	45
Diet cola type, caffeine-free	0	0.0	0.0	51
Diet Slice type	7	0.0	0.0	15
Ginger ale	124	0.0	0.0	26
Grape soda	160	0.0	0.0	56
Orange soda	179	0.0	0.0	45
Root beer	152	0.0	0.0	48
7UP	151	0.0	0.0	10
Slice	156	0.0	0.0	1
Other Beverages				
Cappuccino coffee mix and water, 6 oz	61	2.0	0.0	104
Fruit punch, canned, 8 oz	119	0.0	0.0	56
Fruit punch, local, 8 oz	43	0.0	0.0	50
Hot chocolate mix and water, 1 packet	103	1.0	3.0	148
Hot chocolate, made with whole milk, 6 oz	164	7.0	7.0	92
Swiss mocha coffee mix and water, 6 oz	50	2.0	0.5	36

APPENDIX B
RECIPES

QUICK SALAD DRESSING RECIPES

Thousand Island Dressing

1/4 cup reduced-calorie mayonnaise
1/4 cup fat-free mayonnaise
2 Tbsp catsup
1 to 2 Tbsp minced stuffed olives or dill pickles
1 Tbsp minced onion
2 tsp parsley flakes
1/2 Tbsp chopped green pepper (optional)
1/2 hard-boiled egg, chopped (optional)

Combine the above ingredients and serve over salad greens. Makes about 3/4 cup of dressing.

Nutritional Analysis (per 2 Tbsp): Calories 54, Cholesterol 3 mg, Sodium 300 mg
Percent of Calories from: Protein 1%, Carbohydrate 44%, Fat 55% (3.4 g of fat)

Creamy Ranch Dressing

1 small envelope Hidden Valley Ranch "Lite" dressing mix
1 1/2 cups nonfat or 1% low-fat milk
1/2 cup low-fat mayonnaise (or 1/2 cup low-fat plain yogurt)

Mix the ingredients in a blender or food processor. Makes about 2 cups of dip or dressing.

Nutritional Analysis (per 2 Tbsp): Calories 20, Cholesterol 1 mg, Sodium 210 mg
Percent of Calories from: Protein 21%, Carbohydrate 72%, Fat 7% (0.2 g of fat)

Note: You can modulate the calories and fat up or down by using fat-free mayonnaise or light mayonnaise (with 5 g of fat per Tbsp) instead of low-fat mayonnaise (with 1 g of fat per Tbsp)—or some combination of these products.

Blue Cheese Please Dressing

2 oz blue cheese
1/4 cup reduced-calorie mayonnaise

juice from 1 lemon
1 tsp Dijon mustard
¼ cup nonfat sour cream

Whip all ingredients in a food processor until blended. Makes about ¾ cup.

Nutritional Analysis (per 2 Tbsp): Calories 56, Cholesterol 12 mg, Sodium 161 mg
Percent of Calories from: Protein 21%, Carbohydrate 19%, Fat 64% (4 g of fat)

Note: Fat and calories can be reduced even further by using nonfat mayonnaise.

Vinaigrette Dressing

⅛ tsp salt (or to taste)
¼ tsp pepper
¼ tsp garlic powder
¼ tsp dry mustard
1 Tbsp olive oil
1 Tbsp lemon juice
3 Tbsp apple juice, wine, or beer
1 to 2 Tbsp balsamic vinegar
1 Tbsp olive oil
1 Tbsp red wine vinegar

Combine the first six ingredients and beat well with a wire whisk until
smooth. Add 3 Tbsp apple juice, wine, or beer. Whisk well and add the remaining three ingredients. Whisk well and refrigerate. Shake well before using. Makes about 9 Tbsp of dressing.

Nutritional Analysis (per 2 Tbsp): Calories 60, Cholesterol 0 mg, Sodium 58 mg
Percent of Calories from: Protein 0%, Carbohydrate 14%, Fat 86% (6 g of fat)

BEST BEAN RECIPES

Greek Bean Salad

15-oz can of black beans, drained and rinsed
4 Tbsp seasoned rice vinegar
1 Tbsp extra-virgin olive oil
½ cup chopped red onion
1 cup coarsely chopped yellow bell pepper (or red or green)
   about 3 oz basil and tomato feta cheese (by Churny), finely crumbled
2 to 3 cups fresh basil (or spinach) leaves, washed, patted dry, then torn into smaller
   pieces by hand.

Put beans in medium serving bowl, and add vinegar and oil. Stir to coat beans evenly. Add onion, bell pepper, feta cheese, and basil. Toss well to blend. Makes five 1-cup servings.

Nutritional Analysis (per serving): Calories 180, Fiber 8 g, Cholesterol 15 mg, Sodium 217 mg
Percent of Calories from: Protein 21%, Carbohydrate 46%, Fat 33% (6.5 g of fat)

Simple Tuna and Bean Bake

15-oz can of black beans, drained (about 1¾ cups)
6-oz can of solid white tuna, canned in water, drained
3 celery stalks, chopped
4 green onions (white and part of green), chopped
3 Tbsp parmesan cheese, grated
10¾-oz can of Campbell's Healthy Request Cream of Mushroom Condensed Soup
½ cup light sour cream
4 cups cooked fettucine noodles (or macaroni or similar)
2 to 3 slices less-fat turkey bacon, cooked crisp and crumbled (optional)
4 oz reduced-fat sharp cheddar cheese, grated (1 cup firmly packed)

Preheat oven to 375°F. Toss all ingredients but the cheddar cheese together in medium mixing bowl. Coat a 2-quart baking dish or 9″-×- 9″ baking dish with nonstick cooking spray. Spread tuna mixture in pan. Sprinkle the cheese over the top. Bake for 20 min. Makes five servings.

Nutritional Analysis (per serving): Calories 455, Fiber 9 g, Cholesterol 29 mg, Sodium 581 mg
Percent of Calories from: Protein 28%, Carbohydrate 55%, Fat 17% (8.6 g of fat)

Beef and Bean Tortilla Casserole

1 lb ground sirloin
1 cup chopped yellow onion
15-oz can of black beans, drained and rinsed
½ cup chopped red or green pepper
6 Mission Light flour tortillas
at least 9 Tbsp salsa
8 oz reduced-fat sharp cheddar cheese, grated (or mixture of reduced-fat Monterey jack and cheddar)
½ cup nonfat or light sour cream

Preheat oven to 450°F. Cook beef and onion in nonstick frying pan until nicely brown. Remove from heat and stir in beans and bell pepper. Coat a round 2-quart casserole dish with nonstick cooking spray. Fit one tortilla plus 2 tortilla halves in bottom of dish. Spread 3 Tbsp salsa over tortillas, then one-half of the beef and bean mixture, and one-third of the grated cheese. Repeat these layers two times, with tortillas, salsa, beef and bean mixture, and cheese, except after the last layer of salsa, top with ½ cup non-fat or light sour cream before adding the beef and bean mixture and cheese.

Bake for 10 minutes. Makes six servings.

Nutritional Analysis (per serving): Calories 412, Fiber 7 g, Cholesterol 71 mg, Sodium 548 mg
Percent of Calories from: Protein 36%, Carbohydrate 37%, Fat 27% (12.5 g of fat)

World's Fastest Baked Beans Recipe

8 strips reduced-fat turkey bacon
1 red or yellow onion, quartered then sliced
1 green pepper, chopped
½ cup water, low-sodium chicken broth, or beer
3 15-oz cans of white kidney beans, drained
½ cup yellow mustard
½ cup molasses
½ cup catsup
2 to 3 Tbsp Worcestershire sauce (depending on how hot you like your
   baked beans)

Preheat oven to 350°F. Cook bacon strips on medium-low heat until crisp (not burned). Cut into ½″ pieces. Simmer onion and pepper in skillet with ½ cup water, low-sodium chicken broth, or beer until tender. Combine bacon pieces, onion and pepper mixture, and remaining ingredients in a large casserole dish. Bake uncovered for 25 min, stirring occasionally. Makes ten side servings.

Nutritional Analysis (per serving): Calories 160, Fiber 5 g, Cholesterol 8 mg, Sodium 431 mg
Percent of Calories from: Protein 17%, Carbohydrate 70%, Fat 13% (2.75 g of fat)

Bean and Chili Pepper Salsa

1 cup corn, fresh or frozen (thawed)
2 roma tomatoes, chopped
5 green onions, sliced (white and part of green)
3 Tbsp minced fresh cilantro
5 tsp olive oil
3 Tbsp lime juice (juice from 1½ limes)
¾ tsp ground cumin

¼ tsp salt

1 cup canned garbanzo beans, drained (8¾-oz can)

1 cup canned black beans, drained

½ to 1 cup Anaheim chili peppers (or other mild chili pepper), seeded and finely chopped (use 1 cup if you like it hot)

Combine all ingredients and mix well. Cover and refrigerate overnight or at least 6 hr. Makes about eight ½-cup servings.

Nutritional Analysis (per serving): Calories 117, Fiber 5 g, Cholesterol 0 mg, Sodium 75 mg

Percent of Calories from: Protein 16%, Carbohydrate 57%, Fat 27% (3.8 g of fat)

Salsa Bean Dip

(Also makes a great filling for vegetarian tacos and burritos.)

1½ cups Thick 'n' Chunky mild salsa

½ cup diced onion

2 cloves garlic, crushed or minced

1½ cups canned black beans, drained and rinsed

1½ cups canned pinquitos or white beans, drained and rinsed

½ cup fresh cilantro, coarsely chopped

2 tomatoes, chopped (optional)

Toss all the ingredients together in serving or storage bowl. Refrigerate until needed but not longer than a few days. Serve with low-fat tortilla chips. (There are brands available with 1 g of fat per oz of *baked* chips. The lower-fat *fried* brands contain 6 g of fat per oz.) Makes ten ½-cup servings.

Nutritional Analysis (per serving): Calories 60, Fiber 5 g, Cholesterol 0 mg, Sodium 450 mg

Percent of Calories from: Protein 27%, Carbohydrate 64%, Fat 9% (0.6 g of fat)

TASTY TOFU RECIPES

Teriyaki Tofu and Beef Burgers

1 lb ground sirloin

1 tsp ground mustard (powder)

4 green onions, chopped

⅔ cup Italian seasoned bread crumbs

2 cloves garlic, minced (or ½ tsp garlic powder)

2 Tbsp light Teriyaki sauce

1 Tbsp Worcestershire sauce

10 oz firm tofu

8 hamburger buns
sliced tomatoes and leaf lettuce, for garnish

In medium bowl, mix first seven ingredients until well blended. Add half of the beef mixture to your food processor and blend briefly with half of the tofu. Repeat with the remaining beef mixture and tofu. Form the resulting mixture into patties. Broil until top side is nicely brown (about 8 min), flip over, and broil another 5 min or so until the burgers are cooked throughout. Makes about eight patties. Serve on buns with sliced tomato, leaf lettuce, and other garnish if desired, and low-fat condiments of your choice (catsup, mustard, barbeque sauce).

Hint: You can bake low-fat frozen french fries in your oven at 400°F and broil your hamburgers at the same time.

Nutritional Analysis (per burger with bun, tomato, and lettuce): Calories 284, Fiber 2.5 g, Cholesterol 38 mg, Sodium 465 mg
Percent of Calories from: Protein 30%, Carbohydrate 45%, Fat 25% (8 g of fat)

Tofu and Peanut Salad

about 10 oz firm tofu
½ Tbsp vegetable oil
3 cups bean sprouts
1 small or medium cucumber
3 Tbsp seasoned rice vinegar
1½ tsp low-sodium soy sauce
1½ Tbsp sugar
1 Tbsp apple juice
1½ tsp sesame oil
½ tsp salt (optional)
⅛ tsp cayenne red pepper
2 green onions (white and part of green), thinly sliced
1 cup shredded carrot
¼ cup roasted peanuts, unsalted or lightly salted
2 cups steamed rice, chilled

Cut tofu into ½"–x–½"–x–1" pieces and drain on paper towels. Place these slices on a rack set in a shallow baking pan. Lightly brush their surfaces with oil. Bake in a 350°F oven for about 30 min or until lightly golden on the outside. Set in serving bowl and chill.

While tofu is baking, cook sprouts in boiling water for 1 min and drain. Rinse with cold water, drain, and place in a serving bowl with tofu in your refrigerator. Partially peel cucumber, alternating strips of green for color.

Cut in half lengthwise and scoop out seeds if desired. Thinly slice both halves and add to serving bowl. In food processor or blender, mix together vinegar, soy sauce, sugar, apple juice, sesame oil, salt, and cayenne pepper. Set dressing aside until ready to serve. Just before serving, add onions, carrot, peanuts, and dressing to tofu and cucumber mixture in serving bowl and toss. Makes six side servings.

Nutritional Analysis (per serving): Calories 225, Fiber 4 g, Cholesterol 0 mg, Sodium 75 mg
Percent of Calories from: Protein 16%, Carbohydrate 54%, Fat 30% (7.5 g of fat)

Tofu Enchiladas

7 oz firm tofu, finely chopped
4 oz reduced-fat Monterey jack cheese, cut into small cubes
4 oz reduced-fat sharp cheddar cheese, cut into small cubes
¼ cup finely chopped fresh cilantro, firmly packed
4 green onions, chopped (white and part of green)
2 roma or regular tomatoes, chopped
4 cloves garlic, minced or pressed
1¼ cups canned pinquitos beans (or cooked pinto beans or fat-free refried beans)
8 to 10 corn tortillas
1 cup salsa
1½ cups low-fat bottled spaghetti sauce or tomato sauce
additional cheese for garnish (optional)

Toss first eight ingredients together in medium bowl to make filling mixture. Coat a 9″–x–13″ baking pan with nonstick cooking spray. Heat a nonstick frying pan on medium-low heat. Spray pan with nonstick cooking spray. Add one tortilla. When underside starts getting soft, flip tortilla to soften other side. Remove tortilla to baking pan. Coat frying pan with nonstick cooking spray and add another tortilla. While the second tortilla is warming, add ½ cup of filling mixture to the first tortilla. Roll and arrange in pan with fold side down. Repeat, working quickly until all filling is used (about 8 to 10 tortillas).

Blend salsa with spaghetti sauce (or tomato sauce) and drizzle over enchiladas. Bake, uncovered, for 30 min. Sprinkle tops with additional cheese, if desired, and bake 5 min more. Makes five servings.

Nutritional Analysis (per 2 enchiladas): Calories 397, Fiber 13 g, Cholesterol 24 mg, Sodium 735 mg
Percent of Calories from: Protein 24%, Carbohydrate 47%, Fat 29% (13 g of fat)

Note: If using canned refried beans, instead of tossing the beans with the rest of the filling ingredients, spread about 2 Tbsp worth along the center of the softened tortilla, then add the rest of the filling ingredients. Roll up as usual.

Tofu Teriyaki

14 oz firm tofu
6 Tbsp light soy sauce
1 tsp sesame oil
1 tsp sesame seeds
2 Tbsp sugar
$\frac{1}{2}$ cup + 2 Tbsp apple juice
1 clove garlic, crushed
1 tsp fresh ginger, finely minced (or $\frac{1}{4}$ tsp ground ginger)

Cut block of tofu vertically into about ten rectangular slices. In large measuring cup, blend remaining ingredients to make sauce. Pour sauce into 9"-x-9" baking pan. Arrange tofu slices in sauce. Turn slices over to coat. Broil 10–15 min, then flip tofu slices over and broil 8–10 min longer. Makes about four servings.

Nutritional Analysis (per serving): Calories 135, Fiber 1.3 g, Cholesterol 0 mg, Sodium 779 mg
Percent of Calories from: Protein 25%, Carbohydrate 38%, Fat 37% (5.9 g of fat)

Serving suggestions: Serve over noodles (like low-fat ramen soup) or steamed rice, fill pita bread with this tasty tofu, or eat it with crackers or just by itself.

Tofu Meatloaf

9 oz firm tofu
1 to 1$\frac{1}{4}$ lb ground sirloin
$\frac{3}{4}$ cup reduced-fat sharp cheddar cheese, grated
3 Tbsp fat-free egg subsitute
$\frac{1}{2}$ cup rolled oats (or $\frac{1}{3}$ cup Italian seasoned bread crumbs)
1 small onion, chopped
2 Tbsp Worcestershire sauce
1$\frac{1}{2}$ Tbsp Dijon or other mustard
$\frac{1}{2}$ tsp salt
$\frac{1}{2}$ tsp pepper
3 cloves garlic, pressed
1 cup bottled spaghetti sauce (with no more than 4 g of fat per 4 oz) or tomato sauce

Preheat oven to 350°F. Lightly puree tofu in a food processor. Blend with ground sirloin in a large bowl. Add ½ cup of the cheese; the egg substitute, oats or breadcrumbs, and onion; and the Worcestershire sauce, mustard, salt, and pepper. Mold into nonstick loaf pan (round or rectangular), or similar, that has been generously coated with nonstick cooking spray. Bake 30 min. Pour spaghetti sauce over the top and sprinkle with remaining grated cheese. Bake 15 min longer or until cooked throughout. Makes five servings.

Nutritional Analysis (per serving): Calories 254, Fiber 3 g, Cholesterol 66 mg, Sodium 624 mg
Percent of Calories from: Protein 40%, Carbohydrate 20%, Fat 32% (9 g of fat)

Tofu Breakfast Stir-Fry

2 slices Louis Rich 50% Less Fat Turkey Bacon, uncooked, cut into pieces (optional)
1 cup raw mushroom slices (or other vegetables such as green pepper)
1 cup fat-free egg substitute
7 oz firm tofu (you can lower the fat content further by using reduced-fat tofu), cut into ½" cubes
⅛ cup green onions, chopped
2 cups bean sprouts
Tabasco sauce to taste

Fry bacon in nonstick skillet or frying pan until nicely browned. Add nonstick cooking spray, if needed, to the pan with bacon, then pour in egg substitute. Make scrambled eggs by cooking over medium-low heat and stirring frequently. Add tofu and green onions and cook and stir for a few minutes. Turn off heat. Toss in bean sprouts and add Tabasco sauce to taste. Let rest in hot pan for a few minutes. Makes two servings.

Nutritional Analysis (per serving): Calories 184, Fiber 4.5 g, Cholesterol 0 mg, Sodium 235 mg
Percent of Calories from: Protein 53%, Carbohydrate 24%, Fat 23% (5 g of fat)

Cashew Tofu

6 Tbsp water
2 Tbsp dry sherry
2 Tbsp low-sodium soy sauce (or oyster sauce)
1 tsp sugar
1½ tsp sesame oil
1 Tbsp cornstarch
1 Tbsp low-sodium soy sauce (or oyster sauce)

1 Tbsp cornstarch
1 Tbsp dry sherry
1 Tbsp water
dash of white pepper
14 oz firm or extra-firm low-fat tofu
3 tsp oil, divided
2 cloves garlic, minced or pressed
1 cup mushrooms, sliced, with stems discarded
½ cup sliced bamboo shoots (if canned, drain and rinse before adding)
2 cups snow peas, with ends removed
¼ cup roasted cashew pieces, unsalted or lightly salted

Prepare cooking sauce in small bowl by mixing together the first six ingredients. Set aside.

In a medium bowl, combine a Tbsp each of soy sauce, cornstarch, sherry, and water and a dash of pepper. Add tofu pieces and gently toss to coat. Heat 2 tsp oil in large nonstick frying pan or wok. When oil begins to heat, add garlic and stir. Add tofu pieces and stir-fry for about 3 min. Remove tofu and any sauce from pan and set aside, leaving pan on the heat.

Add remaining tsp of oil. When oil is hot, add mushrooms, ¼ cup water, and bamboo shoots. Stir-fry for 1 min. Add snow peas and stir-fry for about 2 min, adding a few drops more water if pan appears dry. Return tofu mixture to pan. Stir in cooking sauce and cook, stirring gently, until sauce bubbles and thickens (about 1 min). Sprinkle cashew pieces over the top just before serving. Makes four servings.

Nutritional Analysis (per serving): Calories 515, Fiber 4 g, Cholesterol 0 mg, Sodium 405 mg
Percent of Calories from: Protein 15%, Carbohydrate 63%, Fat 22% (12.5 g of fat)

BIBLIOGRAPHY

Ahmed, F. E. Effect of nutrition on the health of the elderly. *Journal of the American Dietetic Association,* volume 92 (9), September 1992.

Alternatives to hormone replacement. *Harvard Women's Health Watch,* volume 1 (2), August 1994.

Armbrecht, H. J. Changes in intestinal calcium absorption and vitamin D metabolism with age. *Current Topics in Nutrition and Disease,* volume 21: 171–199, 1989.

Bailey, L. B. The role of folate in human nutrition. *Nutrition Today,* volume 25 (5), October 1990.

Berger, J., et al. Relationship between dietary intake and tissue levels of reduced and total vitamin C in the nonscorbutic guinea pig. *Journal of Nutrition,* volume 119 (5), May 1989.

Blumberg, J. B. Changing nutrient requirements in older adults. *Nutrition Today,* volume 27 (5), 1992.

Chandra, R. K. Nutrition and immunity in the elderly. *Nutrition Reviews,* volume 50 (12), 1992.

Chauhan, J., et al. Age-related olfactory and taste changes and interrelationships between taste and nutrition. *Journal of the American Dietetic Association,* volume 87 (11), November 1987.

Chumlea, W. C., et al. Fat distribution and blood lipids in a sample of healthy elderly people. *International Journal of Obesity,* volume 16 (2), February 1992.

Cutick, R. Special needs of perimenopausal and menopausal women. *Journal of Gynecological Nursing,* March/April 1984 (supplement).

Dairy Council. Vitamin D—new perspectives. *Dairy-Council Digest,* volume 61 (3), May/June 1990.

Dawson-Hughes, B., et al. Effects of calcium carbonate and hydroxyapatite on zinc and iron retention in postmenopausal women. *American Journal of Clinical Nutrition,* volume 44 (1), July 1986.

DeBruyne, L. K. Nutrition and the aging brain. *Nutrition Clinics,* volume 3 (6), December 1988.

Durnin, J. V. G. A. Energy metabolism in the elderly. *Nestle Nutrition Workshops Service,* volume 29: 51–63, 1992.

Dwyer, J., et al. Maximizing nutrition in the second fifty. *Clinics in Applied Nutrition,* volume 1 (4), 1991.

Estrogen: Putting it into perspective. *The Johns Hopkins Medical Letter,* volume 5 (12), February 1994.

The estrogen question. *Consumer Reports,* September 1991.

Feldman, E. B. Dietary intervention and chemoprevention. *Preventive Medicine,* volume 22 (5), September 1993.

Ferraris, R. P., et al. Regulation of intestinal nutrient transport is impaired in aged mice. *Journal of Nutrition,* volume 123 (3), March 1993.

Flynn, M. A., et al. Aging in humans: A continuous 20-year study of physiological and dietary parameters. *Journal of American Cellular Nutrition,* volume 11 (6), December 1992.

Folk, C., and Powers, J. Nutritional concerns in the elderly. *Southern Medical Journal,* volume 85 (11), 1992.

Food and Nutrition Service. Nutrition and aging. *Nutrition Update,* 3: 1–12, 1991.

Freeland-Graves, et al. Dietary recommendations of minerals for the elderly. *Current Topics in Nutrition and Disease,* volume 21: 3–14, 1989.

Garewal, H., et al. Oral cancer prevention: The case for carotenoids and antioxidant nutrients. *Preventive Medicine,* volume 22 (5), September 1993.

Garmbrell, D. Management of hormone replacement therapy side effects. *Menopause: The Journal of the North American Menopause Society,* volume 1 (2), 1994.

Greenberg, E. R. Retinoids or carotenoids: Is there another choice? *Preventive Medicine,* volume 22 (5), September 1993.

Greger, J. L. Potential for trace mineral deficiences and toxicities in the elderly. *Current Topics in Nutrition and Disease,* volume 21: 171–199, 1989.

The HRT decision in four (not-so-easy) steps. *Women's Health Letter,* volume 1 (1), May 1994.

Hosoda, S. The gastrointestinal tract and nutrition in the aging process: An overview. *Nutrition Reviews,* volume 50 (12), December 1992.

Hosoya, N. Nutrient requirement of the elderly: An overview. *Nutrition Reviews,* volume 50 (12), 1992.

Klein, S., et al., Nutritional requirements in the elderly. *Gastroenterology Clinics of North America,* volume 19 (2), 1990.

Kurzer, M. Diet estrogen and cancer. *Contemporary Nutrition,* volume 17 (7), 1992.

Lieverman, H. R., et al. Aging, nutrient choice, activity, and behavioral responses to nutrients. *Annals of the New York Academy of Sciences,* volume 561: 196–208, 1989.

Meredith, C. N. Dietary measures to decrease disability in elderly women. *Nutrition and the M.D.,* volume 19 (1), 1993.

Meydani, S. N. Antioxidants and the aging immune response. *Advances in Experimental Medical Biology,* volume 262: 57–67, 1990.

Meydani, S. N. Micronutrients and immune function in the elderly. *Annals of the New York Academy of Sciences,* volume 587: 196–207, 1990.

Meydani, S. N. Vitamin/mineral supplementation, the aging immune response, and risk of infection. *Nutrition Reviews,* volume 51 (4), April 1993.

Mukhopadhyay, M., et al. Protective effect of ascorbic acid against lipid peroxidation and oxidative damage in cardiac microsomes. *Molecular Cellular Biochemistry,* volume 126 (1), September 8, 1993.

Over 50? Chances are you need more vitamin D. *Tufts University Diet Nutrition Letter,* volume 8 (4), June 1990.

Pryor, W. A. The antioxidant vitamins as pharmoprotective agents. *Pennington Center Nutrition Service,* volume 3: 25–37, 1993.

Russell, R. M. Changes in gastrointestinal function attributed to aging. *American Journal of Clinical Nutrition,* volume 55 (6, supplement), June 1992.

Russell, R. M. Micronutrient requirements of the elderly. *Nutrition Reviews,* volume 50 (12), December 1992.

Timmons, K. H., et al., Quick and easy steps to a high fiber diet for the elderly. *Journal of Nutrition Education,* volume 23 (5), 1991.

Vellas, B. J., et al. Diseases and aging: Patterns of morbidity with age. *American Journal of Clinical Nutrition,* volume 55 (6, supplement), June 1992.

Walford, R. L., et al. Dietary restriction and aging. *Journal of Nutrition,* volume 117 (10), October 1987.

Young, V. R. Macronutrient needs in the elderly. *Nutrition Review,* volume 50 (12), December 1992.

Zhao, X., et al., Diet and bone density among elderly Chinese. *Nutrition Reviews,* volume 50 (12), December 1992.

INDEX

263